FOR —
ARNETTE & LEN

10-19-95

Warm and caring friends.

May you both tap into a stimulating foreseeable future!

Maurice Krasnow

It's Never Too Late to Have a Future

Adding Life to the Later Years

Maurice Krasnow

VANTAGE PRESS
New York

FIRST EDITION

All rights reserved, including the right of reproduction in whole or in part in any form.

Copyright © 1995 by Maurice Krasnow

Published by Vantage Press, Inc.
516 West 34th Street, New York, New York 10001

Manufactured in the United States of America
ISBN: 0-533-11219-2

Library of Congress Catalog Card No.: 94-90389

0 9 8 7 6 5 4 3 2 1

It is with deep feeling that I dedicate this book to the seniors who contributed to my presentation

When Henry Wadsworth Longfellow was well along in years his hair was white as snow, but his cheeks were red as a rose. An admirer asked how he was able to keep so vigorous and yet has [sic] time to write so beautifully. Pointing to a blossoming apple tree, the poet said, "That tree is very old, but I never saw prettier blossoms on it than those it now bears. That tree grows new wood each year. Like that apple tree, I try to grow a little new wood each year." Longfellow knew the secret of remaining young was developing new interests.

—James C. Humes
Speaker's Treasury of Anecdotes About the Famous

Contents

Foreword ix
Preface xi
Acknowledgements xxi

I.	**Threads of Living**	1
	Incidents in My Life and the Means I Employed to Overcome Them	1
	Expressing Feelings and Emotions	6
	Benefits of My Highest Values	8
II.	**Social, Volunteer, and Employment-Related Activities**	13
	Physical Activities	15
	Volunteer Activity	19
	Employment	24
	Senior Centers	26
	Effects of Stress	27
	More Senior Activity Benefits	29
	A Call to Action	30
III.	**Personal Interests and Hobbies**	32
	Vernon: His Interests and Hobbies	32
	Hobbies	35
	Learn from Living—Live from Learning	38
	Motivation	40
	A Matter of Vision and Hearing	43
IV.	**Adversity**	46
	Adversity in U.S. History	46
	Effects of Adversity	47

	Jean: The Way Her Life Took Shape and Her Responses...	49
	Gus: How He Handled Privation	51
	Growth Comes from Struggle	54
	Turning to Others for Support	54
	Further Respondent Comments........................	60
	Accepting a Challenge When Handicapped	61
	Circumstances..	61
	Coping Mechanisms	62
V.	**Family, Friends, and Lovers**	64
	Mildred: The Benefits of Her Contacts and Relationships..	65
	Spiritual Values	68
	Developing Closeness	70
	Communication..	71
	Reaching Out	73
	Feelings of Insecurity..	75
	Grief and Family Attitudes	76
	Loneliness	77
	Off-Setting Loneliness.......................................	77
	Touching	79
	Love and Affection	81
	Romance and Sexuality.....................................	83
	Different Forms of Love	88
	Life Satisfactions...	91
VI.	**Personal Values**...	93
	The Manner in Which Values Take Hold	94
	Changing Values at Retirement Age	97
	Jim: The Varied Influences and the Coping Mechanisms in His Life	98
	Respondents' Values	103
	Are We Prisoners of Our Past?	105
	Believing in Ourselves: Enlisting Certain Values	105
	Vital Thoughts in Shaping One's Values........	108
	Effects from the Negative Side of Life	109

	Changes and Their Effects	110
	Specific Values Respondents Mentioned	111
	Further Ways Values Can Influence Us	111
	Discarding Some Values and Taking On New Ones	112
	Perspective	113
VII.	**Mental Health**	114
	Our Mental Attitudes	116
	Thoughts Shared by My Respondents	118
	Activity Adds to Health	120
	Nutrition	123
	Further Use of Capabilities	125
	Having a Purpose	127
	A Mental Attitude: Believing in Ourselves	127
	How We Can Have More Control of Our Lives	129
	Pausing Briefly to Reflect	130
	More on Attitudes	133
	Three Final Comments on Well-Being	133
VIII.	**Seeking Gains in Ourselves**	134
	Seeds of Maturity	135
	Some Ways to Carry On	137
	The Importance of Remaining Open	138
IX.	**In Summary**	144

Bibliography 151

Foreword

Our society is changing. It is getting older. We are living longer and staying healthier. We are also more ethnically, culturally, and socially diverse. In fact, the increasing diversity of the older population has become very apparent to gerontology researchers, sociologists, policymakers and others. Perhaps there may have been a time when we could generalize about the needs and experiences of the few persons who reached advanced age because these individuals possessed unique traits and characteristics. Today, the older population is a reflection of our total society as more and more individuals are making the transition into "old age." As such, the need to develop role models has become increasingly important to older persons.

Making the transition from "young" to "old" can be very exciting or it can be very traumatic. Some of us consider this transition as the beginning of a new life. Others feel "finished" and fall into despair. Many older persons worry about the uncertainty of the future and what their lives will be like after retirement. Maurice Krasnow, in his book *It's Never Too Late to Have a Future: Adding Life to Later Years,* addresses this need for reassurance and inspiration. Not unlike our younger years, when we searched for and found examples of success among our peers, so, too, in our older years we can look to "survivors" among our cohorts for motivation and encouragement.

Maurice Krasnow has considerable experience working with senior persons, and as an older person himself, he has been a participant in the changing nature of our country's aging population. He has used his vast experience and understanding to write a book that, in his own words, carries the message "don't give up!; don't feel inadequate or helpless," giving this book an exhilarating and uplifting quality.

He combines his personal knowledge and expertise with that of other older persons to provide us with a book rich with inspirational anecdotes and useful information. Maurice Krasnow said that he wanted to write a book that would motivate older adults today and show younger adults way of having a more productive life in later years.

He has done just that and we owe him a debt of gratitude.

Jorge J. Lambrinos
Director
Edward R. Royal Institute for Applied Gerontology
California State University,
Los Angeles

Preface

Many years ago, I decided that some day I would like to be helpful in improving people's outlook and, in turn, making their lives more liveable. It did not matter whether these were people I met in a work situation or those who may one day read my writings. Thus I became interested in public services in the form of social work and the study of sociology. Social work offered me a means of relieving the problems of those with whom I was involved. I turned to the study of sociology to learn more about people and their behavior. In my middle years, I obtained a B.A. and an M.A. in sociology, with a specific focus on older adults.

Careers in social work and gerontology, the latter in a county office dedicated to improving services for our older population, brought me in considerable contact with these people. As a social worker and senior citizen coordinator for a number of years, I had ample opportunity to meet and deal with retired people. My background enabled me to reach out to these seniors and gain insight into their feelings about life. I was interested in the qualities that made older adults move forward and not give up.

Social studies contributed to my many insights into difficulties that people face with increased age. Retirement and health problems are but two of the changes that older people must accept; yet I became vitally interested in preretirement planning. I felt that education regarding retirement problems could be beneficial to many older adults, so I led discussions on retirement planning. Delving into the adjustments made by older adults became a preoccupation. To study their reactions to such changes, I concentrated on persons in their individual environments.

There is a growing interest today in learning about the concerns and thoughts that inspire older Americans, as well as older generations in other countries. Older people respond in many different ways to change. My focus is on ways that seniors adapt to change and how the flexibility of some interviewed in this book can give food for thought to others. The examples they provide may stimulate us to explore ways we can find satisfaction in our own lives. The essence of the matter is not only how to survive but how to get along, how to renew our lives.

This book is intended to give people courage to improve their outlooks and make life more rewarding and stimulating, particularly for those already retired. My book shows that no one is alone. In privation and disappointment, there are sources to turn to for help. There is hope, and there is no need to ever think of giving up. When we pause to assess what we have, we make inroads into the realization that we are neither inadequate nor hopeless. There are many reasons for carrying on, for living. Finding ways to instill more confidence, to heighten one's self worth, and to lend more dignity to living are the cornerstones of this book.

Most people, regardless of age, want to be self-reliant, especially the present generation of seniors, who have survived frontier life, world wars, and depressions. Because the focus in today's society is on youth, older people often feel a sense of rejection. They feel a loss of power. But freedom to think, speak, and act need not be relinquished simply because of age. Seniors possess qualities that may be valuable to each other and to the greater society as well. Their wisdom needs to be given more opportunity to surface. Our nation can ill afford to place older adults on the shelf and force them to drain the economy.

More thought need be given to ways in which society can assist retired people in remaining productive. A more conscientious support system has already begun. All aspects of aging are now being considered in research centers dealing with geriatrics and gerontology throughout our country. Modern science has enabled people to live longer. The findings of various studies pertaining to the impact of longer life spans is timely and significant. Other countries, also interested in these phenomena, are adding to our overall knowledge. The next step is to find ways to improve the quality of the older adults' extra years. The answers lie with the seniors themselves. Their accumulated wisdom represents a rich heritage.

The chapter headings were formed from answers my respondents frequently gave. (I will discuss my theme questions shortly.) At first, I was overwhelmed by the variety of answers, so I set up many categories. As there were duplications, a weeding-out process followed, resulting in the following chapter headings: Threads of Living; Social, Volunteer, and Employment-Related Activities; Personal Interests and Hobbies; Adversity; Family, Friends, and Lovers; Personal Values; Mental Health; and Seeking Gains in Ourselves.

Many older people today display mental and emotional fears. There is a tendency to live in the past, a nostalgia for the good old days. They see the present as too uncertain. Feelings of apathy prevail. What should be done about this? A large segment of the older population feels frustrated, sad, useless, isolated, and lonely. Feelings of rejection are common. Relationships with children are often quite limited. Fear of old age is widespread. Some are apprehensive of the future, seeking organizations or individuals who can help. They need someone who will listen.

Certain myths and stereotypes are continually generated about older people, but they consist of judgments and attitudes that have no sound basis in reality. One of these myths reflects attitudes many younger people have that older people are not open to new ideas and have a tendency to live in the past. I have found that many older people are open to new ideas and are flexible in their thinking toward the future. D. Elton Trueblood in ''The Blessings of Maturity,'' a chapter from the book *The Courage to Grow Old,* states:

> One of the most common misconceptions about old age is the supposition that it is always a period of intellectual decline. While, for some, decline undoubtedly occurs, this is by no means universal. . . .

My book gives accent to the need for more recognition of the human experience of aging. This applies to the expressed feelings of older adults, reflecting their concerns and aspirations. Stereotypes will diminish considerably with increasing courses offered in gerontology by a greater number of schools in this country. Colleges and universities are becoming more involved in aging research.

More than ever before, considerable material is now being written about people, about their convictions and aspirations in their advancing years. Examining the framework of those years—the things that make people productive, and the things that hold them back—can benefit all members of society.

I made no attempt to shape the contents of this book into a scientific research project, coming to a hypothesis or presenting statistically significant information. Possibly, a research study could be developed from the variables generated in my book; however, my only intent was to offer my readers viable ways to "keep going." Thus, appropriately, the key questions that I presented to older adults over the years were, "What keeps you going? What factors have motivated you and added to your years?"

The theme "What Keeps You Going?" has rarely been touched upon in writings dealing with older adults, and thereby sets this book off from the others. Because of this theme, this book lends itself to reducing wasted lives, gives the reader help in facing life, and carries the message: Do not give up; do not feel inadequate or helpless!—in all, giving the book an inspirational quality.

Too little is known of the encouraging attitudes held by many older adults. Too frequently we do not get close to what older people actually feel about "keeping going." Gaining their confidence made it possible for me to secure their expressed statements.

Their responses have significance because their lives, to some degree, have been reshaped since their days of gainful employment. Even a good number of the women had experienced some form of employment. I was certain that sharing their outlooks with others would give them much pleasure. I asked myself, How might readers improve their functioning by observing the thoughts of other senior adults? The answer is, By improving our scope of practical knowledge.

With few exceptions, most of the persons interviewed for this book were past sixty-five years of age, ranging up to eighty-five (a few past ninety). They came from practically every socioeconomic level. Of the 250 people interviewed, most were middle class and upper-middle class. Interviews took place before and after my retirement. Names of seniors given are fictitious to protect the privacy of my respondents.

In one segment, as a social worker, I made home visits to clients on the Supplementary Security Income (SSI) program. I made contacts at senior centers, senior information and referral centers, adult educational classes, and a senior camp setting. I also contacted personal friends. I derived personal benefit in learning what these older adults had to say.

Most of my respondents have a fairly strong image of themselves. This strong self-image helps them make choices in what they want. It appears that many of their successes in making adjustments are a carryover from their earlier lives.

Along with including my seniors' one-liners relating to "What Keeps You Going," I have included some of their longer remarks. In the first chapter I, too, reflect on my own early influences and experiences in what has kept me going. Also, in different chapters there are a number of "thumbnail" or brief life-sketches of certain seniors' experiences and outlooks. Their comments illustrate the focus of the book.

The book's framework deals with the transition of retirement and the period that begins *after* one retires. Is there a let-down after retirement that causes people to feel less valuable? We need to learn more about what goes into the *adjustments made* at this point in time. *To fill the disturbing gaps* that follow work separation can be a serious problem for many seniors. Some succeed while others do not, but increased leisure time demands adjustments. This problem needs exploring at greater length.

In our society, insufficient guidance is given to the person of retirement age. Too frequently seniors are put adrift with scant information from the companies by which they are employed. Too many seniors frequently have limited insight into coping in a retirement setting. Some have physical complaints, which result in mental problems. Yet the tenacity to keep going is more far-reaching than is generally believed.

Some older people show vitality and determination. Life to them is a dynamic process where movement and action thrive. This can be physical or mental. They find life has something to offer. Many of my respondents have taken responsibility for managing their lives. They try to keep their independence, in spite of the fact that they were not always successful financially. Their responses reflect courage and perserverance. Their secret is based on experience and wisdom.

In the sections of the book where I have presented thumbnail sketches of retirees (highlighting more details of their lives), many consistencies are reflected:

1. Many radiated confidence from an early age.

2. They worked at having a positive attitude.
3. They had loved ones in their midst and/or emotional support from family members.
4. They engaged in varied pursuits.
5. They kept an interest in people and things. (Remaining interested proves to be a key to vitality and well-being.)
6. Their activities continued into their older years especially in terms of services rendered.
7. They were able to adapt to change.

Activity, courage, perserverance, faith, self-confidence, compassion and love for others, and a positive mental outlook are all part of the framework that makes these seniors feel life is worth living. More seniors' life experiences need to be brought to the surface, to be seen on the printed page and read. Older adults have usually experienced deep, emotional turmoil, pain, sadness, and many types of problems. Yet many of them keep going, leading full and active lives. They are happy and hopeful. Many possess a deep inner peace that seems to spring from a sense of self-satisfaction.

It is refreshing to observe that many older adults have a philosophy—a feeling of purpose in their immediate lives that represents a ''keep going'' attitude. Interwoven in this framework is the older person's need to have an interest in *something*. Most of my respondents were people who appreciated themselves. Feelings of self-esteem were evident to varying degrees. Any number of my senior contacts reflected having unlimited resources (some which remain untapped). It is vital that their attitudes and outlooks be passed on since they may be characteristic of many older Americans.

What attitudes do many seniors employ to keep from drifting and wasting their remaining years? What more can we do to learn from our setbacks, our adversity, our pain? How can we have better control of our lives? What are ways to keep occupied? Answers are forthcoming in this book.

Looking inside oneself is simple and can be very beneficial. My thesis is a stimulus to draw out hidden attributes among older adults of retirement age who have lost a grip on themselves and some degree of satisfaction. Many strengths lie dormant within older people. They need to use these strengths to aid themselves in developing better control of their lives, and, in turn, to reduce the impact of stressful situations.

I do not wish to see senior citizens placed on the scrap heap of injustice in our present-day world. I hope to see them shine in their own light and make contributions to themselves, as well as to those about them, in this dynamic world. In various ways I hope to stir more older adults into action, into feeling there is more to live for and more fulfillment as it relates to the future.

The thoughts, ideas, and spirit that carry these respondents forward can be educational material for those who work in aging-related fields. Paraprofessionals can find the book useful in counseling older adults. The manuscript can implement improved services for older adults by its overall insights. It can pave the way toward improved retirement planning, a phase of senior citizens' lives which has been sadly neglected.

In an article in *U.S. News and World Report,* dated December 3, 1990, a reference is made to Robert Coles, psychiatrist: "Coles is fascinated by the survival instinct of older people and wants to find out what keeps them going. . . . '' However, much of his interest over the years has been in understanding young children.

Younger people could be drawn into the ideas and thoughts set forth in my book even though the contents are aimed at older persons, retirees in general. The manuscript lends an orientation to younger age groups in how to live life in terms of improved productivity in the later years. Concepts regarding the aging process should be readily taught in secondary school curricula. Younger age groups should learn more about our nation's older generation. It is significant for these younger people to appreciate how their grandparents and older adults generally are handling their daily lives. Also, sons and daughters below age forty-five need to better understand their own parents who are getting up in years. The topic is universal in its implications.

In this effort, my determination to enhance the lives of those who do not speak up has at long last been brought to fruition. I turned seventy-eight about the time this book was near completion. The time spent with these older adults has added much to my life. I have gained immeasurable satisfaction and pleasure in passing on their thoughts and feelings. I hope that I will strike a chord within the lives of some people with the thoughts that are generated in these pages. I want to imbue the reader with an added spirit—to encourage more hope and faith. I want seniors to learn to feel good about themselves. I wish to inspire in my readers a renewed interest in the future.

Acknowledgements

I wish to pay my respects to those seniors who contributed to the contents of this book. Most will never know how useful and informative their input was. I would also like to acknowledge those kind people who helped me over the years with thoughts, suggestions, and inspiration, adding conviction to my purpose. To these few counselors, including counselors of senior centers and other senior facilities, I owe a debt of gratitude. Ann Morgan Barron, Ph.D., a pioneer in the field of gerontology, who exemplified much to me as a teacher and who, in those early years, gave me significant encouragement in my growing interest working with senior adults. I mention her again in these pages. Harold T. Diehl, Ph.D., one of my sociology professors, contributed considerable guidance in my interests in this field. I refer to him again in the book. Joan Thompson, a counselor and director of a senior center, helped smooth many bumps relating to my personal life, which improved my outlook. Rev. Frank Nelson was a close friend in the later years, one whom I could easily relate to. I discuss some of his senior activities in the book. My sister, Bertha Lasky, who recently passed away, added much to my purposes over the years. She contributed to my well-being perhaps more than I'm able to express. Milton Tepper, a dedicated senior volunteer for many years with the U.S.C. Andrus Gerontology Center and currently an officer on the Los Angeles Commission on Aging, has shared facets of my writing, assisting in giving more clarity to my purpose. Bebe Hineser, a close friend of many years, has been my sounding board for numerous ideas, along with her readiness to offer suggestions; Della Farren, for her concientious editorial assistance; help with typing by Lena Fleischer during the manuscript's final stages; Joe Denhart, for permitting me to use his meaningful teachings; Newcastle Publishing's Kelley Younger, who read the manuscript and expressed many constructive critical comments and suggestions; Patricia Busillo, a guiding light whose capable editing and depth of helpful suggestions contributed more purpose to my efforts in the final stages of this book; and especially to the late Peggy Hayden, for her efforts in motivating me, her help in clarifying my thoughts and her guidance in the actually setting up of this book.

I wish to express an important sentiment relating to Edward Roybal, former Los Angeles, California, congressman, now recently having the Edward R. Roybal Institute for Applied Gerontology at California State University, Los Angeles, named in his honor. In my interest in the field of gerontology, Mr. Roybal always impressed me with his dedication to our seniors. It is most fitting to mention the symbol he has represented to me, having added to my motivational outlook in the aging field.

Overall, in reflecting, I feel we are far from being alone in our efforts to improve what we desire and seek for ourselves, and for humankind about us.

Chapter I
Threads of Living

Incidents in My Life and the Means I Employed to Overcome Them

I am no stranger to adversity. Poverty was the setting for my mother, my sister, and me. Feelings of persecution and depression assailed my mother. The environment in which I lived helped make me become introspective. Many hardships at an early age had a deep impact on me and created a need for me to find ways to keep going. Thus evolved the theme of this book.

When setbacks and privation come early in life, a deep sensitivity develops. In my case, this sensitivity has remained throughout all my years. My background enhanced my ability to cope as an adult. The lack of family love and the taste of poverty started me on a quest of trying to lend more clarity to my existence. Feelings of rejection assailed me; I lived in an emotionally disruptive setting. My future seemed dismal and vague in those early years.

Events of my family life affected me greatly. My parents divorced when I was seven. Before the divorce, I was placed in an orphanage for about ten months (together with an only sister). Later, in the custody of my mother, there was little to help me feel secure. When I became too disruptive, out came the strap. My father was totally absent after the divorce. He made no effort to contact his children. (Through the interest of an uncle, my sister and I met my father again when I was eighteen.)

I was forced to leave high school after one semester in order to obtain working papers. My mother gave me no encouragement to even continue in night school; she saw only the need for me to support the family. It was painful to terminate my schooling since formal education was extremely important to me then, as it has continued to be throughout my life.

True, the early existence of many youngsters parallels my experience. Yet such hardships can certainly scar lives. Why did I not succumb to the feeling that life was hopeless and catastrophic? There are many reasons. Adversity only pushed me to fight harder and not accept defeat. Negative experiences contributed to my knowledge—my experiences were factors in teaching me about the human condition.

During those formative years, the emotional turmoil made me inquisitive. The desire to gain knowledge became an obsession. The trials I endured urged me on. There was always a seriousness within me, a searching, a tendency to reflect. To learn and to gain an insight and an understanding of life were my primary motivating forces.

I visited the libraries frequently. Books were my friends. Compared to my limited and unpleasant home environment, books offered me both companionship and sustenance. I was absorbed with the study of history, English literature, travel, adventure and biographies. All these readings provided a broad education. I felt that I had to learn or else go under—I wanted to survive. The hard knocks were a stimulus. Being forced to depend upon myself developed my interest in education. Enrollment in evening courses became routine.

To compound the disturbing feelings of not being able to continue school like my friends, I found the work experience frustrating. For me, there were very limited opportunities to follow selected fields of interest such as journalism and the sciences. At times my spirit was dampened; at others, it would rise. Illnesses and hospitalization spurred me on to overcome the setbacks. I was not going to allow anything to break me.

The general bickering with my mother and the constant negative vibes caused me to make friends mostly with adults. Reaching out to others allowed me to meet people with some measure of success who imbued me with more hope and confidence. From them I got the feeling that I was not alone. These contacts and the quiet and penetrating talks I had with these people gave me inspiration and improved my thinking. Later in life, I began to realize that, in her own way, my mother had made certain small contributions toward my upbringing. For example, to some extent my mother was a role model in reading and keeping abreast with world news.

Another involvement which benefitted me a great deal was my participation in the Boy Scouts from age thirteen. Exposure to the Scout ideals and tenets brought much well-being and hope to my immediate world. Through the generosity of church board members, I enjoyed a week in camp for two separate summers. This gave me a mental boost that is close to my heart to this day. Yes, we are indeed influenced by the events in our early lives.

While in a carriage, as a baby, I was not always shaded from the sun. This resulted in the need to wear glasses as a child. A strabismus condition (the inability to focus simultaneously with both eyes) developed at age twenty-one. This condition made me very self-conscious because the crossing of my eyes affected my appearance. I was left with emotional scars, but this difficulty eventually made me realize how fortunate I was, and enabled me to deeply appreciate my eyesight. After seventeen years of coping with this condition and the resulting mental stress, the Veteran's Administration performed a successful operation which corrected the problem. This operation changed my outlook on life immeasurably. Further feelings of security resulted. My self-worth rose. I was most thankful.

Four and one half years of military service was also a distinct factor in shaping my life—it began seven months before Pearl Harbor and ended after the war was over.

I was drafted at age twenty-eight. With a strabismus eye condition, some hearing loss, and a recurrent inguinal hernia, I was classified 1A. Apparently, the physical aspects placed me in the Medical Corp and kept me stateside. I was at one point alerted for overseas duty after Pearl Harbor, but the order was rescinded for several of us.

I took medical lab training. I was asked to be a medical observer to an autopsy of a service man, a casualty in one of the maneuvers prior to Pearl Harbor. The setting left a deep imprint upon me in terms of the precariousness of life, making me feel humble in mind, and giving me a deeper appreciation of life.

Wartime military service was a far-reaching experience. We had a grim war on our hands. I felt that I was living on borrowed time. Some of my medical buddies serving overseas never got to return.

I gained *self-discipline.* The word *cooperation* developed plenty of meaning for me, as did the word *responsibility.* These traits became a part of me as time passed.

I had the need of a second inguinal hernia operation midway through this wartime service. Before my military release, this condition recurred for a third interval, bringing about a service disability.

Having had past experience in watch and clock repairing, I requested, about a year before the war ended, to be placed in some kind of precision work. Not long after, approval was given for my transfer to an electronic development lab in the Army Air Corps. In charge was a physicist with whom I much liked working. My inquisitive nature suited me well to this work, which included assisting in setting up apparatus and handling details. (At the time, I had less than two years of high school.)

I had a strong need to direct myself. From the service, I came away with more inner strength and determination to reach some kind of goal through education in the years that followed. The drive I had had all through my earlier years to keep learning continued. Receiving government educational aid during my matriculation was most meaningful and helpful.

At the time of my military release I went on to complete the high school requirements for college entrance. Later, veteran's counsneling guided me in plans for higher education. My wife, whom I married midway through my time in the service, was in accord with me to consider this move. She had much belief in me.

An extremely traumatic event occurred later in my life—my first wife died under tragic circumstances after eighteen years of marriage. Losing her was exceedingly painful. She was a helpmate in so many ways. I was left in a depressed state for quite some time, but the memories of her love, caring, and devotion have given me much faith and inner strength. Friendships and the caring of my two sisters (one being a half-sister who came into my life later) have also been vital assets.

My experiences, both good and bad, have added more purpose and deep feeling to my existence. This has been the case since those early days. I have received many compensations for having gone through these various privations. For this reason, I believe my know-how in the field of aging puts me in a position to help people in many walks of life. I desire to improve the quality and longevity of the senior adult's life.

Expressing Feelings and Emotions

It is characteristic of me to jot down feelings that preoccupy me from time to time. They generate some guidelines for me to follow and assist in clarifying my thinking. These notes were written in intervals of my sixty-eighth year:

> I can have much to say about what I want out of life. Added confidence is a factor along with strong convictions, believing in my successes, daring to take chances, seeing more

security patterns, not being afraid of myself, cultivating warm feelings about myself, and resolutely feeling that I can make changes in my life.

I feel that I have the *power* to make changes. I am not afraid to take a stand and I know that I can lend pleasure and good to other people's lives. I can further say I am finding ever so much good in living by enjoying the 'now' as never before, by not allowing any reservations to enter into the friendships I now have, and by being true to myself.

Much of what I'm exposed to is rubbing off on me these days. In turn, much of what is now me is psychologically passed on to whoever relates to me.

I am assimilating more of life's treasures by looking more into myself. I want the fetters to go. Allowing more good to come out is the key. I want to unmask the hidden fears and the feelings of unworthiness. There is going to be more tranquility within me. I have more power to take charge, to radiate more confidence. Feelings like this come from the depths of me; nothing is rehearsed.

It is imperative that we believe we can change our ability to function better. The old, staid attitudes that I feel about myself have got to go. I feel less fearful of tackling a new way of thinking. Something quieter within now overcomes me. . . .

At age seventy-eight, I expressed:

Not only do I have a concern to develop my inner security, creativity, and progress, but also to promote more understanding of our fellow men and how they can improve their own functioning and creativity. Fulfillment of our diverse needs inwardly and outwardly should be our fundamental concern toward a happier life.

More recently, I made this note:

It's meaningful to communicate my experiences in life. These experiences touch on feelings, emotions, concerns, aspirations, purposes, and strong felt wishes. It takes in what I want from life, and what I want to give to life. It's as though it is a duty for me to feel this way.

Benefits of My Highest Values

Tenacity

Sometimes discussing our personal strivings and concerns with a good friend gives us more security in our own values. Holding fast to old associates can be beneficial.

The experiences in my life influenced my determination to become educated and to find a vocation to my liking. This determined spirit also filled many gaps in my adult and senior years. We need to believe that we can succeed wherever our interests lie. Having purposes promotes tenacity. Essentially, tenacity has existed in most of us in our earlier years in the form of learning and seeking a formal education. The desire to learn remains with many of us, never to be relinquished.

In certain stages in my life I developed a strong will not to have anything daunt me. I developed a persistence and determination to obtain solutions to a problem. In our older years, persistence and determination can continue in our lives.

Tenacity can be a sticktoitiveness in something we like to do, continuing with a strong purpose. By expressing a firmness in something we believe in, we develop further inner strength. Tenacity can turn into a coping mechanism in our older years. It can also be beneficial in aiming for a further purpose or goal, regardless of age. A solid and persistent interest and spirit has to be there. There should be nothing to deter us. These feelings should be laced with gumption—a kind of toughness—courage, and boldness.

Collaboration

One of my greatest assets is that I have always enjoyed collaborating with people and trying to learn from them. I enjoy discussing with others in a group ways to bring about improvements on certain issues or projects. The key is to encourage more understanding. There is much to learn when ideas and thoughts are expressed in a group setting, in joint activity. Here, there is much pleasure in being a participant.

Collaborating is a means of exchanging views or working together on a subject, as in a literary work. It is enjoyable to cooperate with others in producing something. What's wrong with adding your "two cents' worth" in a group setting, expressing your ideas on a certain subject you feel strongly about? This can result in a sense of fulfillment, especially when the subject or discussion is close to you. Participation is healthy when you have some points to offer. Collaborating has its benefits because you are contributing to further understanding.

Collaboration was always important in my life. Involvement in problems relating to people, specifically when I was in social work, came from my need to "connect" with others. Community activity gave me a strong incentive to discuss specific problems with others. This incentive continued in my community work in the field of aging. By collaborating, I learned more about issues and became more proficient and helpful.

Inquisitiveness

As we age, inquisitiveness is a healthy trait. Children possess a natural curiosity, but many people, as they become older, lose it. Fortunately, this trait has remained with me through the years. I am a "bug" for details and sifting through something step by step, always open to reasonable deductions.

My inquisitiveness has enabled me to develop good handcoordination, making me fit for various kinds of trade work. Also, inquisitiveness gave me interests in adventure stories, exploration, pioneer living, cultural anthropology—to name only a few areas. I had a strong curiosity about "roughing it" outdoors (something I eventually explored in great detail). I love man's ingenuity, his adventurousness in searching for artifacts.

Privation boosted my interest in the social sciences, paving the way to matriculate in the field of sociology. Social behavior became uppermost in my mind. My inquisitiveness made me a "doer," adding to my desire to think, to be useful. Being curious, inclined to ask questions, eager to learn, can benefit us all. We might become more proficient in music, art work, or writing some personal history of our lives, the latter a possible gift for family members. Eagerness to learn can stimulate many kinds of ideas and purposes. It might bring about a desire to be helpful to children in different walks of life. Being inquisitive can open up avenues for new hobbies and instill an added outlook. Inquisitiveness makes little room for negative thoughts. Essentially, inquisitiveness can counteract feelings of insecurity.

Openness

The word *openness* means much to me. I used to hold back out of anxiety and fear, but now I have learned to be more open, more direct, in my daily experiences with people. There is more "light" in my life as a result. I like being open to views and convictions. This can involve new ideas and feelings. I desire to expand my horizons.

To you, my readers, I wish to add that openness adds to a willingness to keep learning and gaining new perspectives. Openness involves courage and the ability to look truth in the face, to change our perceptions if necessary. Openness is typical of children, and can be a fine quality to carry into late adulthood. The results can be most beneficial, physically and mentally. Current research points to openness appearing as a factor, to a certain extent, in promoting longevity.

Openness is also a fine trait in a love relationship. I find that by giving love, I am made more aware of feelings. As Theodore Isaac Rubin in his book, *Real Love,* expresses: "The simple truth is that openness begets openness. There is no substitute for it. It is often irresistible."

Communication

Efforts to foster human understanding begin with communication, making it a priority for many seniors. Much can be accomplished by sharing concerns with people, family. Educational settings and political affairs are examples. Verbal and non-verbal communication are both significant; they stimulate thought. Being a good listener is also essential to developing improved communication.

I hold the communication value as one of the most important ones in our lives. I am giving communication expanded coverage and feel it more appropriate to discuss this value at length in my chapter "Family, Friends, and Lovers."

Chapter II
Social, Volunteer, and Employment-Related Activities

> Older people are making their voices heard in politics, education, the arts, consumer affairs, environmental and pollution problems, legal matters, safety and crime, and welfare.
> —Julia Braun Kessler
> *Getting Even with Getting Old*

Activity is a significant need among older people. Seniors desire to be active, to have some involvement, whether it be conversational or physical. They look for things to spark their interests.

They need and enjoy reaching out to others as they had throughout their younger lives. Duties and obligations were paramount over the years; they can describe in detail the many chores in which they were engaged. Responsibilities in past years have challenged and strengthened the older person, and this needs to continue as a primary, motivating force.

Inactivity, lethargy, and apathy are negative behaviors the medical profession warns against, and for good reason. These traits are detrimental to a person's health and well-being. Inactivity can result in anxiety and depression, but exercise can relieve these problems.

People wear out more from *in*activity than from activity. Bertrand Russell stated it well when he said:

> I am convinced that survival is easier for those who can enjoy life, and that a man who has sufficient vitality to reach old age cannot be happy unless he is active.

Studies have shown in the past several decades that the busiest people are the happiest. In a workshop run by the Ventura County Department of Mental Health (California), the leader stated that activity is a very important facet of life for older adults.

An insight relating to preparing for the inevitable slowing down process is well-expressed by D. Mechanic in his article, "Social Factors Affecting the Mental Health of the Elderly":

> Older persons tend to be less physically strong, slower in response, and more cautious and concerned about responding correctly but may counterbalance these with more mature judgment and broader experience . . . .

Mature judgment and broader experience are helpful in senior peer counseling and supportive rap groups. Seniors support one another in self-esteem groups and in the loss of spouse groups. Their broad experiences also help solve community problems and help them counsel children and teenagers.

At another point, Mechanic expresses:

> Inactivity is a significant risk factor for the deterioration of the elderly, and one of the significant preventative insights

that can be derived from the literature is the importance of encouraging continued functioning. . . . It is through continued activity that individuals maintain their skills and sense of social value.

Many people think about what they'll do when they retire before they reach retirement age. When you ask yourself what keeps you going, you should also ask what incentives you have in your life. What brings you satisfaction? What is it that makes you tick? Most often the answer will focus on some kind of activity or involvement.

In some instances, my respondents mentioned as many as a half dozen or more categories that contributed to their longevity and positive outlook. Other areas of involvement include keeping abreast of current social problems, government and political affairs, and local and county matters. The outer world can have an impact on the older person. Seniors should be well-informed.

Physical Activities

Walking is an important, valuable activity for seniors. An eighty-two year old I observed had great enthusiasm and spoke of having "lots of get-up" for her age. To maintain good health, she takes regular walks and is generally quite active—physically and mentally. Understandably, walking as an exercise, in many situations, needs to be prescribed by one's doctor. There are many pluses gained from walking; one of which, notably, is that it increases the heart's efficiency. Harry, age seventy-three, who was previously into sales work, repeatedly said to himself as he took his regular walks, "Better than the pills, better than the pills. . . . "

An eighty-nine-year-old lady bowler who had begun bowling at age sixty-five expressed: "I enjoy the exercise and the game. And it's a social thing for me. I never get bored with it. Well, I do get bored when the ball doesn't go where I want it to." Today there are many senior bowling groups. If a person has some agility and enjoys camaraderie, this kind of activity can be beneficial and much fun. A few inquiries at a bowling center can easily place one on the inside track relating to such bowling groups.

Going on trips or vacations has significance in the lives of older people, adding to their adjustments and well-being. Picture another example of activity as seen on TV. A man was celebrating the fiftieth anniversary of his first climb in the Grand Tetons (up a mountain that is 13,700 feet high). This man, now seventy, had been a mountain climber for many years. I felt awed by his stamina, his nerve, and his courage. His friends spoke of him as a man of order and harmony. When he had reached the summit, he had experienced feelings of respect, admiration, and love toward those who had accompanied him on the climb.

"I might wear out, but I'll never rust out," is a popular expression. In one setting where this was stated seniors were competing in athletics. There is even a Senior Olympics which is gaining popularity throughout the world. Founded in 1969, the group's motto is "Living Youthfully."

At an older adults' camp outing during a recent summer, I had the experience of taking a hike with a group. This was in the mountains at 4,000 feet. We came upon a lovely waterfall. Looking down on the rustic setting 40 feet below, we could see the base of the falls, which were about four feet wide with a narrow path leading to the base. I had previously traversed this difficult, steep pathway, strewn with boulders, to the bottom. On the present occasion, two of the women in the group, both about sixty-five, decided after some hesitation to hike down with me. These sturdy women, with my assistance, handled the rough hike in a most efficient manner and were exhilarated by their efforts. They had given themselves permission to do something challenging. The two women later told me they felt that this experience was the highlight of their trip.

In the retirement years I have become attracted to the Sierra Club, a nationwide organization. Some walking tours are geared for those who cannot do strenuous walking. The hiking composition varies much in length and terrain. Many older and retired persons participate in this fine outdoor activity. Sierra Club chapters are listed in phone books nationwide. You can also obtain this information from Parks and Recreation departments.

James C. Hume, author of *Speaker's Treasury of Anecdotes About the Famous,* has an anecdote about Henry Wadsworth Longfellow on the subject of activity as follows:

> When the poet Henry Wadsworth Longfellow was well along in years, his hair was white as snow, but his cheeks were red as a rose. An admirer asked how he was able to keep so vigorous and yet has [sic] time to write so beautifully. Pointing to a blossoming apple tree, the poet said, "That tree is very old, but I never saw prettier blossoms on it than those it now bears. That tree grows new wood each

year. Like that apple tree, I try to grow a little new wood each year." Longfellow knew that the secret of remaining young was developing new interests...

The late Dr. Paul Dudley White, in *Getting the Most Out of Your Fifties,* made this meaningful observation:

When one reviews the histories of people in their eighties or nineties and over 100, he finds that the very great majority have been physically and mentally active persons throughout their entire lives.

An excerpt of a report prepared by the Soviet Union's Institute of Gerontology ties in with Dr. White's statement. They say, "The more the brain and muscles are used, the less they age." The Institute also asserts that the steadiness and consistency of physical activity over the years, from early youth to the older years, prolong life.

A change of pace can give a person a lift. Activities that are physically and mentally stimulating include things like an extensive trip, trying one's hand at photography when on a journey, meeting and conversing with people for the first time, or seeing the process by which some item is made. The main objective is to get away from the commonplace and to jolt oneself out of a rut by a new setting once in a while. *Why not?*

Any number of older people have the ability to say, "I choose to do," and to find new vistas. One simply needs to find things to do that one is able to do and that are enjoyable.

It is plain that activity appears to promote improved physical health. The older person's mental alertness seems to improve as well. Activity brings about a buoyancy, a trend toward making more friendships, and an inclination to be happier. When we are activated into something we enjoy, an inner peace develops.

Volunteer Activity

When we feel quite self-contained and satisfied with ourselves because we like ourselves more, we tend to reach out, desiring to do some good. This ''good'' could perhaps be in the form of volunteer work—to be of service in some manner. Below, I have provided some resources you may wish to contact for volunteer activity.

The Peace Corps

The Peace Corps is an excellent way to avoid feeling retired. There is no upper age limit for the Peace Corps. Various stipends are given for employment, and Peace Corps benefits are available. A retired mechanical engineer who had a membership with an affiliated committee on aging whom I came to know joined the Peace Corps, putting his skills to use in a foreign country. He spent a year in this service. The enthusiasm and satisfaction he expressed from this experience was easily seen.

In the pamphlet, ''Senior Volunteers in the Peace Corps,'' a volunteer, Odi Long, age eighty-one, observed: ''When you have idle moments when your mind is not occupied, you start feeling your age. I don't have idle moments.'' The same pamphlet states:

Older Americans often desire a channel through which they can share their work and wisdom. There is a need to demonstrate the ability to do a good job in a most productive manner and to make a contribution.

The Peace Corps has seventeen area recruiting offices nationwide. Listings are in the white pages of telephone directories under U.S. Government. The main office is:

Peace Corps
Recruitment Office
806 Connecticut Avenue NW
Washington, DC 20526
Toll Free: 1-800-424-8580, Ext. 93

The DOVES Program

Another kind of activity is the DOVES Program. A brochure states:

The program provides the schools with carefully selected and trained senior citizens to supplement the work of classroom teachers. Assistance is given to elementary and secondary school students contributing to their achievement, self-image, interest and motivation. Seniors can be helpful in tutoring groups or individuals, helping in the classroom or library as clerical or recreational assistant. (Also) sharing career or job experiences, reading or telling stories, counseling and more.
   The program was cited for its recognition of the valuable resources senior citizens and retirees can bring to the education process in ever increasing variety of ways.

This brochure also states that the DOVES (Dedicated Older Volunteers in Education Services) Program received national recognition in the Spring of 1977 from the National Center for Voluntary Action in Washington, DC.

In the Los Angeles, California area, contact:

The Volunteer and Tutorial Programs
Los Angeles Unified School District
450 North Grand Avenue, Room G-252
Los Angeles, CA 90012
Phone: (213) 625-6900

The DOVES program is involved nationwide. A branch of DOVES includes schools and communities and has an information network for volunteer programs. This includes various programs in education and finances among others. This organization is called:

National Association of
Partners in Education
209 Madison Street, Suite 401
Alexandria, VA 22314-9820

Retired Senior Volunteer Program (RSVP)

RSVP has an extensive file from which to choose for people who are interested in participating in volunteer work. Some areas they can refer you to include: senior multi-purpose centers, hospitals, schools, Planned Parenthood, community service centers, and mental health clinics, to mention a few.

The Retired Senior Volunteer Program is funded by the Action Department of the Federal government. In the San Fernando Valley of Los Angeles, the main address is:

Retired Senior Volunteer Program (RSVP)
8134 Van Nuys Boulevard, Suite 200
Panorama City, CA 91402
Phone: (818) 908-5070

The Foster Grandparent Program

For those who like children there is a national, government-sponsored program, started in 1965, called the Foster Grandparent Program. Older adults volunteer their services to interact with needy children for which they receive a small stipend and countless other benefits such as love, being needed, and the satisfaction that comes from giving. The potential benefits are numerous.

Excerpts from a survey on volunteering entitled, "How Being Helpful Helps the Elderly Helper" are worth referring to:

> The volunteers "reported more life satisfaction, self-esteem, will to live, and less depression. . . . This would suggest that encouraging elderly subjects who are in reasonably good health to help others in some structured program could lead to a better overall quality of life for those who do."

One of my interviewees, James, age seventy-two, remarked: "Living is a reality here and now, in the present, not something in the past or in the future. If we can do something for our fellowman, do it now." James takes much interest in people; a friend of his informed me he works with the blind. James said that he stands on his ideals and principles, and he likes to keep active.

While I was a guest at a senior citizen nutrition program, a woman over seventy entertained everyone by playing the piano. Her renditions awakened a nostalgia which had a decidedly beneficial impact on the seniors in the dining hall. She demonstrated much talent. A number of the seniors joined in singing to the tunes. At the intermission, she and I discussed many old songs from the musical vintage years of the '20s and '30s. At one point she told me that she is always searching for new music and added that she makes trips away from her neighborhood to find better and more varied selections.

Some older people still do some instructing in art and Bible study, as well as various forms of counseling. Being useful, showing kindness, and helping others are all a means of keeping active. *Giving*—love, advice, babysitting when needed—are all popular considerations among older adults.

Betty, a widow in her early sixties who had been married over forty years said: "I want to have a life again. I had a good life. What is important to me is to be doing something for someone. As long as there is life in me, I'm going to be active. I feel there is something out there that I've never done that I would like to experience—that's my curiosity."

In a well-known survey, "Who the Senior Citizens Really Are," Louis Harris and Associates reflect a significant finding:

> . . . People sixty-five and over are very much alive and well. They decidedly do not view themselves as individuals who

are rotting away... They are not only alive and well, but they have hopes and aspirations toward a better life. They want to be more active and they want to contribute to society above anything else.

Employment

Checking out part-time work with temporary work services is an excellent means to be gainfully occupied after regular retirement. Much depends on the person's concerns and interests. There are some older adults who desire to supplement their income. Others find a dislike in having extra time on their hands.

Currently, there are many companies seeking retirees for part-time work in many parts of the United States. In a most recent book, *Retirement Careers: Combining the Best of Work & Leisure,* DeLoss L. Marsh gives a stimulus in improving our life style during retirement. Marsh asserts that "[t]emporary help services present a quick route to employment. They offer a variety of career opportunities working for different companies . . . ''

National Council on the Aging (NCOA)

The NCOA has been working with the U.S. Department of Labor and community agencies to help older people find jobs, increase their incomes, and learn new skills. Title V of the Older Americans Act is the federal law that makes this possible.

For further information, contact:

The National Council on the Aging, Inc.
Senior Community Service Employment Program
600 Maryland Avenue SW
West Wing 100
Washington, DC 20024
Phone: (202) 479-1200

In the Los Angeles, California area, contact:

The National Council on the Aging, Inc.
2500 Wilshire Boulevard, Suite 402
Los Angeles, CA 90057
Phones: (213) 365-0700 or (818) 837-4346

Second Careers Program

In some localities a Second Careers Program has been established, specializing in services for older workers. The Program is non-profit and remains dedicated to helping mature workers continue being productive. Some of their services are Job Placement, Job Search Assistance, Computer Instruction, and Retirement Planning. In the Los Angeles area, Second Careers is located at:

Second Careers
3923 West Sixth Street, Suite 216
Los Angeles, CA 90020
Phone (213) 380-3166

Some people cannot give up working after formal retirement. Of course, that is one way of never *feeling* retired.

Senior Centers

Ellen, at eighty-eight, still drove a car and was still able to get around reasonably well. The warmth that she radiated was quite contagious. I felt that I was in the presence of a wonderful human being. She informed me that what kept her going and gave her strength and enthusiasm was the senior center near her board and care home.

At senior centers people have the ability to express what keeps them going. Such communication represents a direct way to do away with frustration, apathy, and sagging morale. Their thoughts reflect *action,* which keeps these negative feelings at bay. The *doing* counts and heightens their satisfaction. There is a positive feeling of accomplishment.

In senior centers there are many kinds of activities and classes. Senior centers are more and more representing a vital role in communities throughout the nation. Writing classes, rap groups which raise issues and answers, needle craft classes, and beginning dance classes are only a few of the programs. Travel trips are becoming the vogue in these centers. Many centers now have nutrition programs, serving a lunch at a nominal cost five days a week. Opportunities for volunteer work can fill gaps in an older person's life. Some centers even have shuffleboard and billiards.

At the 1990 National Council on Aging, "Networks," U.S. Commissioner Joyce Berry made these observations:

> Many older persons' lives have been saved by the senior center. Some may think such a statement is dramatic, but it is true. Many older persons build their lives around the local

senior center. That's where their friends are, that's where the information is provided, and that's where there's love. . . . [Senior centers] can help fill the gap by providing information and access to services that some older persons need.

Senior multi-purpose centers are a literal godsend. They represent a beacon of life, a place to turn to when hope is dim, a means of counteracting an otherwise lonely existence. (I have had the pleasure of participating in men's discussion groups as well as in mixed groups at various centers.) The rapport among seniors here can contribute to our well-being. The gains are abundant and well-recognized. There are many social and recreational services available for seniors. One merely has to make inquiries and be willing to participate.

Effects of Stress

Some stress is a normal part of living and cannot be controlled. Some stress can be favorable to our lives according to health research. The amount of stress that each person can absorb varies. It's the way we respond to stress that makes a difference between health and illness.

Some tensions and pressures are frequently present. They can drive us and give us incentive. The pressures can be put to good use. But I would be foolish to try to convey an image of an overwhelming number of seniors who are well-contained and radiate exceptional confidence and exuberance. Interspersed among older adults are those whose lives are filled with sadness, insecurity, and loneliness.

Many haven't the physical ability to put their knowledge to use.

Multiple factors shape the ability or inability to cope in the later years. Low self-esteem from an early age prevents some seniors from making adequate adjustments. They continue to find it difficult to gather their inner resources. The complexities of modern culture compound the problem.

Many people today fear close relationships. Morals are lower. Feelings of frustration are often economically oriented, and there is considerable pessimism about the future. People are afraid of giving in to alcohol and drugs or losing their mental faculties; some are even fearful of taking on responsibility.

People's lives are less structured today than several generations ago. Formally, there was more tranquility, cohesiveness, and family orientation; families were less dispersed. Communication among family members was more frequent, and the mass media played a less significant role. Segments of our older population are being affected by these negative factors.

Admittedly, seniors have varying strengths and abilities to propel themselves forward. Inertia is deadly. Seniors must demonstrate a will to go on and to not give up; they must generate a strong will to live.

Counteracting excessive stress can be accomplished by tension-releasing methods such as sharing feelings with a relative or friend; involvement in hobbies or interests that are enjoyable and productive (a discussion on hobbies will follow shortly); exercise of different kinds, wherein walking has many benefits; developing relaxation techniques—one can manage a stress situation by relaxing mentally for brief intervals; focusing on volunteer work, and looking for new challenges. Taking control of your life is a means to deal with stress.

In a final thought on this subject, Dr. Hans Selye, one of the outstanding authorities on stress has stated: "Man should not try to avoid stress any more than he would shun food, love, or exercise."

More Senior Activity Benefits

In what is called the Marriott Senior Living Services Volunteerism Study of April 1991, the percentages that gave major reasons for volunteering among volunteers sixty-plus years old were:

Helps others	83%
Feels useful	65%
Moral responsibility	52%
Social obligation	30%
Companionship	25%
Loneliness	17%
Uses spare time	15%
Learns new skills	15%
Boredom	14%
Guilt	5%

In this Senior Volunteer Study, 1,000 people sixty and older throughout the United States were interviewed. The study found that 40 percent, or 15.5 million seniors, who volunteer gave 992 million days of service during the past year. Another 37 percent, or 14 million seniors, are potential volunteers who said they would volunteer their time if they were asked.

This observation by a well-known gerontologist, Robert N. Butler, in his *Why Survive?* is apropos:

> There are many ways to be emotionally healthy in old age, but several common themes emerge: The desire to be an active participant, to make one's own decisions, to share mutual love and respect with others. Healthy older people experience many of the same feelings and responses as people of all ages, yet old age has its own unique flavor. . . .

Dr. Butler succinctly rounds out the essential factors toward emotional health and well-being among older adults.

We should treat ourselves well in life. Our self-esteem rises when we learn to express ourselves more. Speaking of expression in a physical way, some of *my respondents showed they felt better about themselves just by the way they walked—briskly.*

To keep going requires having a certain amount of energy. Almost all the seniors interviewed have had some kind of drive, no matter how small. These people were both mentally and physically active. One interview on television with an eighty-year-old woman posed the question, "What keeps you going?" Her reply was: "I refuse to get old."

A Call to Action

The importance of being productive gives one much to think about. To have many irons in the fire at different stages has value. *Effort* is required. Nothing worthwhile comes easily. We should have an objective, an inspiration, and make an attempt to carry out whatever plans we make. We have to come to terms with what we can do, and do it.

Senior adults' activities should never stop. Their functioning, their striving, should always continue. It follows that caring and reaching out have their own rewards. Yet, activity by itself is only a phase in the whole life of a senior. As we go along, we will turn to other factors which always interact. Overall, we cannot remain static; we have to make ourselves *move*.

Chapter III
Personal Interests and Hobbies

> The quality of a life is determined by its activities.
> —Aristotle
> *Nicomachean Ethics*

Often *the reference to* activity, as pictured by many respondents, did not imply doing things with others. They indicated that they spent time by themselves reading books, cultivating a hobby, working in the garden, etc.

One of my respondents, Vernon, is a good example of someone who remains active through hobbies and interests. I became acquainted with Vernon and his wife during a writing class. Let us look at a brief sketch that shows how Vernon keeps going.

Vernon: His Interests and Hobbies

Vernon and his wife agreed to be interviewed in their home. Although Vernon's wife hardly entered into the interview, I quickly learned that her role has been a most supportive one. Vernon, at age seventy-five, is rather tall and slim in appearance, and conveys a great deal of wisdom. He made me feel that he is a man with much compassion.

"Most of the time my wife keeps me going," said Vernon, married fifty-four years. He touched on his interest in genealogy which was encouraged by his wife ten years earlier. His wife was instrumental in helping Vernon learn about his ancestors. Vernon explained that through his wife's efforts, people in his family "have become more alive to me, instead of being just names and dates in the past."

Finding his grandfather's name in the genealogy section of the Los Angeles Public Library fascinated Vernon. It sparked an interest in a project that grew into a major involvement. "It changed our lives," Vernon said. The vast amount of time he and his wife have spent on this project has brought many rewards. "I became closer to my own family by visiting my aunts and cousins out of state. Our family ties are stronger."

Vernon's wife is a big help to him. He told me that his wife can read rapidly and retain what she reads, an ability he lacks. The research they do together gives their life purpose and meaning.

In addition to remaining active, Vernon places a prime importance on health. "The most important factor in anybody's life is their health," he said. "I have always enjoyed good health—you have to have your health to maintain a good outlook on life. A lot of people enjoy being sick because they can be the center of attention. They get the center stage. Many people have imaginary ill health. It's a big problem. Others don't make an issue of their problems and go on in spite of them."

Among his insights, Vernon feels that we should not become slaves to our television sets. The habit of "watching the bad things that go on in the world—the rapes, the murders, the muggings, etc., limits our ability to function, instilling all kinds of fear in us so we won't even want to go out on the street.'' He believes that seniors need to get out of their houses as often as possible. To him, television should never be more than a fill-in. However, I'd like to add that the television does present many *good* programs. What we need is discrimination in the tuning process.

Vernon points out that the ability to keep going involves ''the desire to improve ourselves—we should always try to learn something new each year, such as a new hobby.'' When I commented on the beautiful stained-glass windows in his living room, Vernon informed me that they had been one of his projects about ten years ago. They were *his* achievement. He had taken a course and spent thirty days designing and completing the project. At the time of completion, Vernon gave himself a party, inviting seventy-eight people to see the finished product.

Before retiring, Vernon was never greatly interested in art. Nevertheless, some of his landscape paintings were framed on the walls, attesting to his ability. He claims that he never did anything artistic prior to these efforts except to dabble in photography. In recent years, Vernon has taken up woodcarving and clay sculpture. He has produced some fine pieces which would do credit to a museum exhibit. He has also instructed others in these pursuits.

Vernon's wife sat quietly through the interview, content to have her husband be the spokesman. But at one point she interjected, ''I don't want you to think there were only roses. We had many hardships.'' Her husband immediately added, ''Adversity challenges and builds your character.''

This couple gave me the feeling that there was a real closeness, a mutual supportiveness, and a deep love between them. Currently, Vernon and his wife are taking a community writing course at a local college. They wish to register their experiences in life and pass them on to their younger family members. Vernon makes this concluding observation: "People who learn more and seek more knowledge are filling one of man's greatest drives." This reminds me of something I heard a retired doctor say: "Older people should fight isolation by socializing with others and should keep learning new things."

Hobbies

Putting some effort into an activity, like communicating or talking to another person in order to share some problem, forms a basic way to keep going. Motivation of any kind can be a driving force. Occasionally, we are activated by a desire to try something new, like taking a course in school, learning a new language, or pursuing a new hobby.

Seniors wish to continue being resourceful and to apply the talents they have. Some outlets are cooking, crocheting, knitting, and needlepoint. Many men and women find gardening and driving a car enjoyable. Frequently, there is a strong incentive to cooperate with other seniors, and even other age groups, in certain hobbies. Both sexes desire to remain productive and useful in some way. This is a challenge.

Many seniors speak of "something to hang on to" that helps them through each day. Others express a need for diversions, a way to spark their routine. This includes listening to music and sports; becoming a member in an older adult's club; affiliating with churches, fraternal organizations, and the like.

As a hobby, calligraphy is popular today. With practice, a person can develop a personalized kind of lettering and handwriting. This can be very satisfying and relaxing. Many senior centers now have classes in this art form. The hobby can set in motion a perspective for other kinds of art enjoyment.

Creativity and an active imagination are good traits. Creativity reflects growth and productivity. Creativity can encompass many activities and is a good trait to have in exploring new paths. These could be outdoor painting, interior design, flower arranging, writing, and music of all kinds. Imagination ties in with creativity. With imagination we try to create new images or ideas by combining previous experiences. We sometimes attempt to learn to appreciate the imaginative creations of others, especially works of art and literature. A retired man I know is learning to bake bread. His wife, who is still employed, finds in him a real helpmate. All these activities can be enjoyed in groups and not only on an individual basis.

On "Over Easy," the TV program about older adults, an eighty-five-year-old man had taken up weaving. Prior to his new hobby, he had developed pains in his hands. He began weaving on the advice of the National Arthritis Foundation. Combining creativity, interest, and exercise, this craft allowed him to remain active, control his arthritis, and to function better. The man had formerly been interested in ceramics, but his arthritis interfered. The weaving was an activity he could still participate in and enjoy.

Roy, a warm and friendly man in his late seventies who I met several years ago, was involved in two hobbies. He kept a vegetable garden with many kinds of vegetables and skillfully crafted wood clock-frames of several sizes. One of his uniquely framed clocks graces an end table in my home.

A retired couple, Jim and Dorothy, friends of mine who live near the Idaho border in Oregon, told me what keeps them going: Jim, nearing sixty-five, built their ranch houses himself and felt it was a form of pioneering. The couple took much pride in starting from scratch and ending with the houses completed. With much pride the husband exclaimed, "Ah, to see things built!"

In discussing the significance of age, Gertrude, who was eighty-seven, explained: "I keep busy; there's lots in that. I do the best I can. My children are good to me." I asked Claire, eighty-five and currently a nurse's aide, what keeps her going. She replied, "Work." Nellie, an eighty-eight-year-old who has lived many years on a farm, expressed that her long life was due to "outdoor life—chasing cattle, pigs, chickens and children."

Rose, in her mid-eighties, said one way of adjusting to the older years is to "continue in the stream of life and to prod oneself gently into the activities one can still do." Tom, age seventy-one, tells us: "If you're bored with your life today, you'll be bored when you're old. If you're interested, active, and alert, you'll continue to be that way."

Laura, age seventy-four, mentioned that she has memberships in several social organizations. She says, "I work and play. I'm busy all the time. My secret in reaching old age is to keep busy, to get involved. I've always been active; I get involved with others.... To have the joy of this moment. The present is what is important.''

In most instances, people held nine-to-five jobs for a long time. After mandatory retirement, a person can retire to something more enjoyable. Avoid *feeling* retired. Mandatory retirement is one thing, but the matter of *feeling* retired is another. Sometimes childhood interests can emerge, influencing you to revive some heartfelt activity at the retirement age. One of my respondents took this stand: ''No one with sound mind and body should ever retire, regardless of age or money.''

Learn from Living—Live from Learning

Making an effort to learn and gain new insights adds value to the retirement years. Continued learning can add to the quality of leisure time. Today there is a trend for older adults to enter into further learning. One has only to visit senior multi-purpose centers, for example, or note the adult education classes in various parts of the nation to see the picture. An insight comes from the United Way Strategic Institute's July-August 1990 publication: ''Colleges and universities will increasingly recruit older Americans (aged 65 and older) as students.''

Some years ago, I attended an adult education course where I became friendly with Bill, an eighty-three-year-old. When I was driving him home one day, he made this observation: ''All my life I've been a student. I try to study now. I try to study people. My hobby is people. If I can't do them any good, I can't do them any ill. I believe that when you're 'harmless,' no harm can come to you. If you are a help to people, they will be a help to you.''

"You have to have something to hang on to," said William, past seventy. He spoke of "a trickle of understanding" which he feels is *not* called wisdom. He continued, "I look at life realistically. I look at life with a sense of humor. It all depends on what demands you put on yourself. Your mode of thinking and observation has a lot to do with it."

Mary mentioned reading a lot and having a keen interest in the political scene. She said that these concerns have been on-going all her life. "I'm never too sick. I've learned to take care of myself," she added. She is eighty-nine.

Beatrice, age eighty-four, told me that she spends hours a day studying. "Most people quit studying when they get out of high school," she said. "The older part of your life can be the most lovely part. To love other people, to give to other people, gives you more security, but you have to earn it."

While on an auto trip, I chanced to meet a gentleman named Robert in a restaurant. Robert and I struck up a stimulating conversation in which he declared that he had much to live for: the beauty of the mountains, the sunshine . . . "I have love in my heart." The man, past sixty, touched on faith and spirit. "We are here on this earth to do something with our lives. God put us here for a reason." Robert told me that he had once had cancer, but that it had been cured. He feels it essential to have positive thoughts. He has filled the need for something positive with music—not just listening to records, but learning, in his sixties, to play a guitar.

The U.S. Post Office turned out a twenty-cent stamp bearing an excellent axiom—"Learning Never Ends." Apropos to that, a recent newspaper item tells of a ninety-eight-year-old woman who received a high school diploma in Madison Heights, Michigan. The woman declared, "I'm taking more classes next year and I'm going to learn, too, like anyone else can."

Why place limitations on ourselves? Exposure to new events, lectures, and discussion groups can be beneficial. In discussing his longevity at age ninety-one, the late Rabbi Edgar Magnin said, "One of the secrets is to keep learning." A large number of older adults speak of a need to continue to learn from living and live from learning.

Adult education programs can help lend direction. Many colleges throughout the nation and in foreign countries have Elderhostels where courses of many kinds are offered to seniors in a favorable setting, with a chance to live on or near the campuses at a reduced cost. These educational opportunities, plus the chance to socialize and the stimulus to visit new places, are without equal. To pursue such opportunities write:

Elderhostel
75 Federal Street
Boston, MA 02110

A catalogue will be sent to you.

Motivation

Older adults have to direct a conscious effort toward finding avenues to keep interests alive. *Self-motivation* must become a more vital force in generating enthusiasm in their remaining years. Frequently, this was developed in their younger years, but self-motivation can become more difficult and require prodding and direction as the years take their toll. The effort in adding a further skill can help our self-motivation.

One senior expressed feelings of uncertainty. "I'd like to get tied up with something, but I'm not sure how," he said, desiring to become involved in some way. To fill a gap in his routine, he was grasping at ways to be useful. Just vegetating takes away vitality. Incentives have importance in bringing fulfillment. There is a deep satisfaction in placing some good into the *now* and thus into the immediate future. The effort is worthwhile.

A high school play that I once saw had as its theme: "Know what you're looking for and then reach out for it." The strong convictions the young actors demonstrated touched me. I was surprised that young people foster such thoughts, and I was impressed by their ability to place these thoughts in a dramatic form. I felt that this theme should be ongoing throughout a *lifetime.* This reaching-out process has meaning. In going through life, it is good to have a guiding symbol of some kind and to continue the *unfinished business of living.*

A study, "The Effects of Aging on Activities and Attitudes," found that changes in total activities were significantly and positively correlated with changes in total attitudes; those who reduced their activities as they aged tended to suffer a reduction in overall satisfaction, and, conversely, those who increased their activities tended to enjoy an increase in satisfaction.

The key is motivation. It comes in various forms as was shown recently on the TV program, "Real People," where a dance therapist was leading older people in wheelchairs to the music of the "Blue Danube Waltz." They were waving their arms and moving their lips in time with the music. Some of the seniors had lovely smiles. The movements of their arms were reminiscent of butterflies. These older people had various afflictions. A few were stroke victims. However, the dance therapist had no need to force her patients in this activity; the group acted as if it was normal.

I have touched on the significance of stirring ourselves into activity. It appears to me that deep-seated interests grow best when we get involved in the mainstream of life. When seniors (over 700 of them) were given the opportunity recently to attend a dance festival at a large hotel, they were vibrant and happy in the setting. It was inspiring to see so many older people dancing. The event generated great camaraderie; these friendly seniors got themselves involved.

Those of you reading this who aren't yet seniors will benefit from the realization that if you live a loving life, reaching out to others, the gains can be immeasurable in your older years. Good habits don't disappear simply because of advancing age. The ability to keep going in the later years is greatly enhanced by similar efforts at an earlier age.

According to Dr. Arthur Flemming, formerly the head of the President's Commission on Aging, older people continue to have a desire to be involved in life, and do not want to be put on the shelf. Dr. Flemming cited the case of a man, age ninety-four, whose productive life was not over. He quoted the nonagenarian as saying, "My last days will be my best days."

"When I was ten years old, I was considered a little delicate," remarked George, a ninety-year-old who takes care of himself in his own apartment. He smiled after making this observation, seeming impressed with himself, at the same time flicking the ashes from his lighted cigar. I could not help observing that George gave the appearance of a foreign diplomat. A wry smile played on his lips, which did more to explain his attitude toward life than fifty words could have done. It seemed as though he was defying the medical profession by the manner in which he flicked the ashes. I smiled along with him, much impressed. I wish now that I had probed deeper into the secrets of his good health and happiness. I suspect it all came back to attitude. George has an active mind; he was surrounded by a number of books.

A Matter of Vision and Hearing

I'd like to add a few thoughts relating to visual and audio impairment. As I have said, over the years I have had my share of eye problems. As we become older, it pays to periodically receive check-ups. A complete medical eye exam is in order at certain intervals, particularly when a person experiences any change in vision. A visit to an eye specialist, specifically an ophthalmologist, is meaningful. If needed, cataract surgery is one of the safest types of surgery and overwhelmingly successful in restoring vision. An ophthalmologist specializes in cataract as well as other kinds of eye surgery. In various areas of the United States, there are eye referral-centers as well as hospitals dealing with eye problems.

There has been significant advancement in corrective eye surgery and vision research in general. Many medical organizations, such as the L.A. Institute for Ophthalmic Surgery, speak of miraculous breakthroughs in laser surgery, cataract, and glaucoma surgery with the enormous improvements in the treatment of all eye disorders.

Hearing also calls for diligent care. With many older people suffering hearing losses, it is valuable to be checked occasionally by an ear specialist so that hearing adjustments may be made if necessary. As with vision, advancements are increasingly being made in the hearing field. *Longevity* magazine of December 1990 stated that hearing loss is our nation's second leading handicapping disorder, affecting over 30 million Americans.

With a well-fitted hearing aid, I gain much in my limited hearing. I am a member of the organization called SHHH. What is SHHH? Here is the statement from the San Fernando Valley Chapter Newsletter (in the Los Angeles area):

> "(SHHH) Self Help for Hard of Hearing People" is a volunteer international organization of people who do not hear well, and their relatives and friends.
>
> It is a nonprofit, nonsectarian educational organization devoted to the welfare and interests of those who cannot hear well but are committed to participating in the hearing world.

The membership represents various ages and comes from various walks of life. When you have a hearing loss, there is a depth of understanding and a need to reach out to help one another to improve each other's functioning—by conversation, lectures, insights in hearing aid developments, and the like. Inevitably, you feel you have something in common in the atmosphere of such meetings, and this is occasionally coupled with a social gathering of some kind. The national office is located at:

Self Help for Hard of Hearing People, Inc.
7910 Woodmont Avenue, Suite 1200
Bethesda, Maryland 20814

A few of the membership benefits are: a nationwide chapter network (practically every state in the union is represented in the SHHH program); award-winning SHHH Journal; up-to-date information on technology; list of assistive devices; and latest research information.

Allow me to conclude by observing in this chapter that basically, we should do whatever we can to preserve our ability to function. Only by taking an active part in taking care of ourselves can we be all we can be.

Chapter IV
Adversity

He knows not his own strength that hath not met adversity.
—Francis Bacon
Of Fortune

Adversity is, I believe, a significant force in making adjustments. People's lives are frequently filled with crises, obstacles, and handicaps, causing distress and sadness. Problems are a part of living. They beset us all, yet adversity does not have to result in tragedy; it can be a stimulus for personal growth. The choice is ours.

Adversity in U.S. History

Our early pioneers worried about droughts, which affected crops, limiting their food supply. Transportation was difficult, making it a challenge to bring supplies to their remote living areas. They had no telephones for communication and no automobiles; these people relied primarily on horses and wagons. Lighting facilities were primitive. Gaslight and electricity had not yet been invented. Their medical knowledge and supplies to fight disease were limited. In those early days, cooking was done on an open fire in iron pots, and many things were made by hand.

These pioneers were toughened and strengthened by the hardships they faced. They learned to adapt. Their lives were a series of challenges. Discipline and self-reliance were strong values among these people. Their plight was uncertain, and cooperation was necessary to build a future.

Seeing films portraying these pioneers' difficult westward journey toward a new life stirs admiration. We cannot help but identify with their privations and miseries, as well as the care families showed each other. These early settlers carried themselves with worthiness and self-respect. They developed survival skills.

Louis D'Amour, the famous western writer, said,

> "The men and women who lived the pioneer life did not suddenly disappear, they drifted down the years, a rugged proud people who had met adversity and survived . . . a quality that distinguished them was dignity."

Pioneer influences and traditions remain. *The pioneer spirit lives in many of our older generation, never to leave them.* At this point in history, we are most fortunate to gain from the experiences of those who came before us.

Effects of Adversity

People may wonder how adversity can be directly connected to anything positive—for example, to the drive that keeps people going—but sometimes we grow more from adversity than from good fortune. We can actually benefit from suffering, hardship, or misfortune. Usually, in an adverse situation, we *do* something. Crises are almost always a source of enrichment and renewal because adversity encourages the search for new solutions. If something bad happens, then emotional adjustments are necessary, but these adjustments can become a challenge to make one's life more liveable.

Helen Keller, who lived a life of total blindness and deafness, set quite an example. What an inspiration she has been to the world in the way she kept herself going! Dwelling for a moment on her handicaps can stir our minds profoundly and make us appreciate having our own faculties. On the commemoration of Helen Keller's birthday a few years ago, Lawrence McMillan wrote a letter to the *Los Angeles Times* discussing her prolific life. He said, in part:

> The "acute disappointment" of her life was not her total deafness. It was not even her total blindness. Rather, it was her lifelong inability to speak like a normal human being to other human beings who could hear.
>
> Even to this she reacted not only by working hard all her life to improve her speaking voice, but also by giving defeat a twist of inspiration.
>
> She declared it had taught her to identify with the frustrations of all human striving. "I understand more fully," she said, "the infinite capacity of hope." (Copyright, n.d., Los Angeles Times. Reprinted by permission.)

Occasionally, adversity is not a result of one's own hardships, but the result of caring for another who suffers. For example, when a child is born with a handicap, the hardships will be shared by the parents as well as the child.

Jean: The Way Her Life Took Shape and Her Responses

Jean, now past seventy, is of average height, rather plump, wears her hair quite short, and uses no make-up. She usually wears sports clothes and presents a neat appearance. She is a warm, friendly person, making you feel immediately at home in her presence.

Jean was always poor. She was married at age twenty, but two weeks before her wedding her prospective husband lost his job. The first year of their marriage was difficult. Jean desired children but could not have any. Twelve years went by. Her spouse was drafted and spent three years in military service.

In her husband's absence, her parents showed her love. "There was much love in the family—an awful lot," Jean said. She was always sensitive to her parents' needs and was close to them. During the war her father died of cancer, which was very difficult for her.

Jean's husband came home to visit her on furloughs. Then, unexpectedly, she became pregnant. "When I got pregnant, it gave me a wonderful feeling of well-being, a real lift." She eventually had two children, but was forced to raise them alone while her husband was overseas. To help financially, she ran a boarding house.

Jean noted that her son, at age eight, was a loner, keeping much to himself. This deeply concerned her. "I felt stress for the first time," she said. To combat the tension at home, Jean began to volunteer for the PTA and Child

Guidance Association. Later, she became a board and charter member. This volunteer work was important to Jean. She had always placed great importance on work since her first employment over twenty-five years ago. "I loved my job.... They were happy days for me.... I liked working with people."

In recent years, Jean and her husband have been engaged in community activities. "I am grateful to my friends for the ideas they gave, as well as their help in getting me to become involved."

Jean's health has been failing. She now has heart trouble, and for fifteen years has had diabetes. To arrest cancer, she had to undergo a mastectomy. "I easily get stressed, but I am learning how to get out of stressful situations," she said. Reading and attending group counseling for patients recovering from cancer assists her in coping with her problems.

Her outlook? "If you are a person interested in things, you can be a happy person. You *learn* by helping people [her emphasis]. You become knowledgeable, you accomplish more," she said as her eyes sparkled. Pausing a moment, she said with a smile, "I realize that I have led an interesting life, because you are interviewing me." The support she gets from her husband has been a strong influence in Jean's life. He has always been very supportive, and they've continued to have much love between them—"a love you can trust."

When I asked Jean what keeps her going now, besides her positive outlook, Jean answered that many good things have happened in her life. "I'm not finished yet—I want to see a better world. When I see what seniors are going through, it breaks my heart. . . ." She then cited a few examples of senior issues and needs. Jean concluded, "I would like to see the world made better where people do not have to struggle so much and can care for each other. Each time I help others, it helps me."

Adversity had coexisted with many of the good things about which Jean spoke. She became the kind of person she is now through a number of setbacks and much suffering. Crises paved the way for growth. The positives and negatives brought her a depth of feeling. Many factors motivate people to keep going. There is much pathos and drama interwoven into the lives of each human being; each has a story to tell. Here is another.

Gus: How He Handled Privation

Gus, age sixty-five, is slender and well-built. He is above average height and has a cultured, natty appearance. He radiates a quiet and kindly manner. He has not had an easy life, yet he always faced his troubles. He was in the Service for four years during World War II and was stationed one year in London during the German siege.

Incendiary bombings were typical during that time. Regarding the bombings, Gus said, "I felt feelings of terror right down my spine. I gained a real respect for the English, their courage, intelligence, and ability to maintain a calm in very frightening circumstances." He said it helped his own morale to see their stamina and heroism.

Gus was a serviceman with Patton's army during the Battle of the Bulge. With a headquarters' group he "saw people in adversity, in dire circumstances—they didn't despair." Returning home from the Service, Gus felt depressed and serious. "I was physically exhausted—I learned to be humble," he said.

In recent years, a slight limp, caused by polio at age thirteen, became increasingly painful. Gus was forced to undergo hip surgery, which he came through without any permanent disability.

The operation did much to change his life. Looking back he says, "You develop a compassion for people who suffer pain. You become more sensitive to other people." After the surgery, Gus was on crutches for two and a half months. "To be able to take a good, long walk with my wife—to share all the things we are looking forward to. . . ." When he walks, he says he breathes the air consciously.

Months after his hip operation, Gus decided to retire from his work. After retiring, he felt let down; he was very mentally depressed. He said that he was "super-active" all of his life; upon retiring he didn't know "how to fill the vacuum." He relates that he had some prestige while working. He found that a senior citizen's multi-purpose center helped him (particularly a men's support group) to improve his mental attitude.

I asked Gus if he would explain in more detail what he meant by saying, "I learned to be humble." Gus conceded that his humbleness resulted from physical deprivation. He was able to walk even though he was told at first that the hip surgery had a 50-50 chance of success. Without much pause, he mentioned that the war scenes, the death and destruction that he witnessed on the European front in World War II, made him humble. "It made me appreciate each day we have in America. I learned to appreciate all the simple things in life that we take for granted. When I returned to the States, that's when it truly hit me."

Because he decided to attend college after his release from the service, Gus needed money, and was able to save twenty cents a day in carfare by walking a mile to and from the city limits. He said that he made no attempt to put on a front in terms of his economic status. "I was being humble before the facts. Rather than kid myself, I would size up my real situation. I cared about how I spent my money and my time."

During his four years away, he learned his parents had divorced. "They let me down," he said when he learned of the divorce. Later, he found his mother had a brain tumor. She survived, and is still alive at eighty-two, although she is in a rest home now because of a speech impairment and paralysis on one side. Gus said he's always had a good relationship with his parents.

"My grandmother had a tremendous effect on my life. She had much physical privation. I was deeply impressed by her; she always gave me so much of herself to others. She showed us, by example, all the really worthwhile values of life." Gus has used his grandma's values to help him face whatever problems life sends his way. Married thirty-three years, Gus speaks of having a very good marriage, during which he and his wife had three children. "I am very lucky. The first night I met my wife, I became aware of her tremendous kindness. I immediately considered her a buddy. I can see more things to love in her every day. When a man is lucky enough to have a kind and loving wife, he is very, very fortunate. . . . One thing that keeps me going is the deep love that I have for my wife and that she has for me."

But Gus doesn't reserve all his love for his wife. He is never too busy or occupied to take time to communicate with other people. Gus is a warm, feeling human being, with deep sensitivity for others.

Growth Comes from Struggle

We can all point to stressful situations in our lives. It is paramount to overcome the pain and disturbances. Reversals or hardships are usually checked by movement—by *taking action.* There must be a challenge to change circumstances; there must be a wish to bring back some good or hope into our lives. Hope can grow from despair.

A counselor from a group of which I was once a member said, "Growth happens from struggle." There is a lot of truth in this statement. Hardship can be a source of strength for one's ego and self-esteem. In varied situations, older people have expressed that survival skills learned from the Great Depression years had a strong bearing in motivating them toward an improved status in life.

Turning to Others for Support

If we are weakened by adversity, and if we continue to feel discouraged and depressed, a serious situation is obviously made worse. It can be most agonizing when we make no effort to turn to another human being in our distress. Turning to someone, a person who is genuinely interested, is essential. We must make an effort to verbalize the disturbance and identify the emotional pain. Isolating ourselves is the worst thing we can do.

We must ask ourselves: Are we really alone in the world? Is it possible to make our lives more livable? Can we make new friends? Can we turn to a relative who cares? Can we turn to reading, listening and further learning? Can spiritual guidance benefit us?

In a previous chapter, I referred to many kinds of senior center activities. These centers are prevalent nationwide. Bereavement therapy groups for widows or widowers are often available. Individual counseling is frequently offered, as well. Senior centers have information and referral services for specialized kinds of assistance. With all these resources, a painful state of mind can be alleviated. Some such services can be found in the telephone directory under the following headings:

Legal Advice
Nutrition Programs
Church Organizations
Bereavement Groups
Transportation Needs
Alcoholics Anonymous
Al-Anon
Community Centers

Local mental health clinics can also be valuable in times of excess stress or adversity. Many of these clinics are run by hospitals. Many medical centers have senior adult day treatment centers that provide a flexible program of psychiatric services as a low cost alternative to inpatient hospitalization. The emphasis in these programs is to assist the older adult in maintaining independence at home and in the community, and in developing positive coping skills. You can contact a center in the Los Angeles area at (818) 885-5348.

American Association of Retired Persons (AARP) is a worthwhile organization from which you can secure many kinds of information. Throughout the nation, AARP has chapters with varied functions, and many have social import and are excellent means to develop friendships. Local chapters can be found in most telephone directories.

Occasionally, older persons can receive information from government officials, such as their congressional or senatorial representatives. In respective districts, field deputies serve to assist in making such referrals as well.

Bearing on the themes of earlier privations and growth in our lives, Harry W. Hepner, a penetrating writer in the field of gerontology, makes these excellent observations in his book, *Retirement—A Time to Live Anew:*

> Those persons who have learned to deal intelligently with their earlier problems achieve the inner strength and happiness which make for worthy living in the later years. Everyday problems and seemingly unbearable situations stimulate them to acquire insights that eventually enable them to enjoy the experiences that contribute to genuine inner growth. They attain great perspectives . . .

The well-known Maggie Kuhn, founder of the Gray Panthers, made a pertinent statement:

> ... the things that were most difficult and most painful for me to do day by day were the things that have given me strength and have given me a certain insight that serves me well today.

Louise, a woman in her mid-sixties, remarked, "Life can be very cruel, but every now and then I get a lot of joy. This keeps me going. I want to see how it comes out. Just think about all you can accomplish in life." She told me how adversity had affected her nine years earlier: "After my husband passed away, I had very few funds and I was all alone. I couldn't go around crying; I had to make a life for myself. I knew I had to do it and I did it." Louise learned to bowl. She joined a square dancing group, went on group tours, developed more friends, became a committee member in social groups and a coordinator in a senior nutrition program.

Privation and pain, such as losses in childhood, cause many people to feel more deeply. Through learning, striving, and hardships, along with purpose, we can frequently gain strength. Like me, my sister was unable to complete high school. Her life was filled with many hardships over the years. She had begun poetry and short story writing, and worked on developing these talents. She is currently in her seventies, and some of her material has been published in the past few years. Her outlook has expanded in a meaningful way. She said, "I have been blessed with fortitude and the ability to cope."

Seniors Handling Privation

Columnist S. Norman Feingold lists the results of a quiz that appeared in the July-Aug. '91 issue of *The Futurist*. One of the statements on the quiz, "A life crisis often has positive effects," received an overwhelming number of affirmative answers. Feingold states, "Peter Ebersole and Jean Flores of California State University, Fullerton, found that more than 40% of subjects studied said the worst crisis they ever faced had a long-term positive impact, even causing them to alter their opinion of the meaning of life. The authors state that those people who can transcend pain and adversity and look forward to a positive future are not rare."

Kathleen, at the age of eighty-one, was a searching, inquisitive person. The "hardships in life—looking for something better" help keep her going. Life has not been easy for this woman; through the years she's suffered many financial difficulties. She also mentioned that what keeps her going is the "something that's missing." What she means by this is that lack of finances or human contact drives her to seek what she needs. For example, she tries to offset loneliness by meeting people and conversing with them.

Marie (my name for her), at ninety-five, her eyesight failing, attends a college lecture, an introductory course in humanities, once a week. The *Los Angeles Times* described her as follows:

> What matters to her is that she is learning. She says, "I'm basically a nosey person so I want to know more. I'm learning a lot in this course. They ask me, 'How can you go to

school if you can't see?' I tell them, 'If I can see through my ears, I'm enjoying everything I hear.' " This woman was rather familiar with some aspects of the course, having visited Rome and Florence some years ago and seeing the Renaissance paintings being talked about in her class. "I just eat this stuff up," the elderly woman said. "It's like I'm in Italy all over again." (Copyright, n.d., Los Angeles Times. Reprinted by permission.)

Marie's experience brings to mind one of my respondent's words: "Everything sinks in more when you are older. You brush it off when you're younger. In your life you will have weeds, moisture, sunshine and clouds."

Lillian, an eighty-year-old, had experienced tragedy and deep sadness when she lost all five of her children during epidemics years ago. After telling me this, she paused and continued: "I lack an education. The only education I received has been the Bible, my husband, and *Science and Health.*" Lillian explained that learning by these means gave her vitality to cope over the years. She added, "People can't understand why I'm happy—everybody seems burdened these days. You have to build your own inner security to have peace of mind. You have to thank God for your adversities. You stand in your own light." Lillian has gained moral courage and growth by developing inner security. She doesn't consider adversities as tragedies; she sees them as ways to grow.

Many senior adults refer to tragedies and serious physical ailments in the lives of other people. This tends to soften the impact of hardships in their own lives. One respondent who has walked with a crutch for the past thirty-five years said, "We should look at other people worse off than we are." From such a vantage point, a person can appreciate his own ability to cope on a larger scale.

Siegmund H. May, in *The Crowning Years,* asserts that a tragedy can be the beginning of a new awareness and appreciation of life:

> Must we be shocked by a tragedy to discover and use our hidden resources? Probably not. But in some cases it may, as in the case of this man (recovered from a serious heart attack), change one's attitude and, therefore, one's conduct of life.

Negative happenings are a part of living. However, certain negatives in our lives can be turned around, bringing *a change in attitude* (as May points out), but this requires effort. As many in their older years expressed—some of the lack in their lives gave them more determination to withstand the difficulties.

Further Respondent Comments

Grace, age seventy-eight, said, "I had heartaches as well as love—that's why I'm strong." These heartaches related to a long-time problem of alcoholism in her mate, along with the serious illness of her mother in her later years which required Grace's attention. She says that she has always been active and keeps going "because I love life—I am a happy-go-lucky person." Grace has the company of parakeets.

"What keeps me going?" exclaimed Martha, considering the question I asked. "I think back and try to count my blessings, notwithstanding my losses and bitter disappointments, and I'm glad I'm OK—that I still can smile.'' Martha added, ''I count my blessings, like the thirty-five years I had with my husband, who is now deceased.'' One of her disappointments was her pain from the inability to bear children. Another was the loss of her parents at an early age.

Accepting a Challenge When Handicapped

In July, 1981, handicapped climbers were televised ascending Mount Rainier. These fearless people were all smiles after their conquest. Certain kinds of handicapped people can do many astounding things because they are continually challenged by life.

These climbers illustrate that people can accomplish many tasks in spite of handicaps. We all set our own limits. Seniors need positive examples because there is a tendency to pamper ourselves and make excuses for limited movement and activity as we grow older. Some seniors blame everything on age.

Circumstances

Eleanor Roosevelt was a person who felt the economic deprivation and physical suffering of many people of the world. In a book she wrote two years before her death, at age seventy-eight, *You Learn by Living,* she expressed:

> Unhappiness is an inward, not an outward, thing. It is as independent of circumstances as is happiness. Consider the

truly happy people you know. I think it is unlikely that you will find that circumstances have made them happy. They have made themselves happy in spite of circumstances . . . People can surmount what seems to be total defeat, difficulties too great to be borne, but it requires a capacity to readjust endlessly to the changing conditions of life. . . .

Coping Mechanisms

Writings dealing with older adults have given adversity recognition as an influential factor in learning to cope with life. Margaret Mulac, in *Leisure Time for Living and Retirement,* gives us a helpful insight:

Adversity is our school and proving ground. It teaches and tests us. Without it, we can develop neither strength to suffer nor ability to endure. Every time we avoid responsibilities which may cause anguish or pain or employ the tranquilizer method to alleviate it, we deny ourselves the opportunity to practice fortitude and thus increase the limits of our endurance. In failing to face up to sorrow, tribulation, and pain, we diminish ourselves. . . .

When in a quandary, there is a need to change the unfavorable situation. Through stresses and privation, we can go on striving; we can go on to form new beliefs and ideals.

I could say much more about people who maintain a courageous outlook in spite of being plagued with difficulties in their older years. There are any number of seniors who do not give in to their difficulties. They develop a resistance. I have observed that many older adults are drawn closer to each other by their mutual adversities.

Intertwined with our daily tasks of problem-solving are our *values.* We can also speak of them as *ideals.* Adversity contributes to our values. Values are like sentinels as we move through life, silent reminders helping to light the way. An extensive discussion of values is soon to follow in chapter six.

Chapter V
Family, Friends, and Lovers

To love, and to be loved, is the greatest happiness of existence.
—Sidney Smith
Lady Holland:
Memoir of Friendship

Amongst seniors, the need for communication is a deep concern. Many of my respondents indicated the importance of liking people, establishing friendships, and absorbing other people's ideas. Many felt these human benefits have given them much to live for.

"My children are good to me," remarked a woman in her seventies who feels this has been a significant factor in lengthening her life. A number of seniors refer to their children in warm terms and indicate that the relationships they have with their children have definitely influenced their longevity.

A strong sentiment is, "The older you get, the more you want someone who cares." When asked, "What keeps you going?" the first answer by some of my seniors, including one eighty-six-year-old, was "To feel I am needed."

Older people, especially, want to feel needed. To some, *feeling needed is the backbone of their existence.* The value of communication, being asked for advice or an opinion, or even receiving a phone call at regular intervals, cannot be overemphasized.

Being close to a person really helps. As a result, our lives are more livable. Frequent dialogue and honest sharing improve the level of understanding and aid in combating loneliness. However, any attempt to interact with others requires action, showing an interest in another person.

There is much evidence to show that people cannot be totally independent of others. The need is there. *We make ourselves happier when we allow people to enter our lives.* The ability to feel with another person gives us a lift that cannot fully be measured.

Mildred: The Benefits of Her Contacts and Relationships

One of my respondents, Mildred, was a spry, medium built lady radiating friendliness and culture. At seventy-one, she still spoke with a twinkle of enthusiasm when she said, "... An expectancy of good keeps me going. You have a choice and the positive is so much easier to work with." Mildred's unpretentious manner reflected a warmth and sincerity that made me feel as if I'd known her for years.

Mildred was an only child. "I was shy," she said. Her father didn't have a good income, but she was unaware of that. "Mother was very creative, a beautiful homemaker and a skillful seamstress. I was dressed quite well because of my mother's skills. I wasn't aware of lack." She spoke of her parents as genteel, "but from a Victorian background. I received love but not in a caressing sort of way."

In those early years, Mildred's plans for higher education were interrupted by marriage. She had wanted to attend college, yet her parents had not encouraged her. They could not afford to do so. Married at nineteen, Mildred had a real love relationship. She and her spouse were together for fifty-one years. Two children came from this union, a boy and a girl.

Mildred's spouse learned to be a pilot in the Marine Corps. He was a Reserve Navy Lieutenant in the thirties. During World War II he was in the Air Transport Command. His missions were always dangerous. "There was joy and moments of sheer terror," Mildred remembered. Her spouse's work as a pilot kept him away from home a great deal. "We were never bored with each other; I was so tickled to have him home."

When I asked (in the vernacular) if the "sun rose and set in her man," Mildred responded in the affirmative. "He had such a gentle disposition and yet such strength, and he was so kind. Everybody adored him. He was very well-liked." Following his time in the service, Mildred's spouse became a professional pilot with TWA. He spent thirty-five years with them and received a tribute and special recognition at the time of his retirement, having been an early pioneer and having made a contribution to aviation. A fellow pilot once observed about her husband that "his friends were legion and his enemies unknown."

Her husband had passed away eight months before the interview. "I am so grateful for all the happiness I have had and all that I am still expecting," Mildred said. *"It's the position you're put in. How you handle it helps mold the person you finally become. You are a composite. It makes you compassionate and forthright. It depends on where you're coming from and how you accept things"* [emphasis mine].

Within one week of her husband's passing, Mildred said that she decided to return to senior-center activities. "Where would I find people more supportive?" she asked rhetorically.

Volunteer work is not new to Mildred. She was a Girl Scout leader, a Gray Lady in hospitals all through World War II, a volunteer at Red Cross Blood Banks, and has participated in United States Bond Group activities. "I've done volunteer work all my life," she said with a smile. Currently, she is into peer counseling, making home visits to counsel the elderly on various problems. Included in her activities is her work on the planning and fundraising committee of a senior citizens' club. "It's a challenge to keep going," she asserted. "I have been fortunate to have such happiness. We don't know what motivates people. I try to understand them. Life should be joyous." She feels there should be more communication between people. *"I could have easily been passive all my life, but adversity creates necessity and need provides a challenge* [emphasis mine]. It's my decision how to handle it. Time's a-wasting. Each day is so precious."

Spiritual values are important, Mildred feels. "I admire all religions, not what they espouse—it's *how* you live it, *how* you put it to use." She continued, "The wonderful things that are wrought by prayer.... I have been blessed with wonderful friends ... If you give of yourself—that is the main thing. You are enriched." Mildred also told me she follows the Golden Rule.

A TV commentator in a senior citizen public forum once made a reference to what an elderly woman, age 103, wanted—"to be loved, useful, and listened to."

In his book, *On Growing Old,* gerontologist A. L. Vischer made this comment:

> People need to feel that they belong somewhere. And the majority of people get this sense of belonging from their family and from their work...

Having various kinds of friends adds luster and stimulus to our immediate world. Friends create a motivation to keep moving; they give life added meaning.

Often we have fears which prevent us from establishing friendships. We feel vulnerable and afraid of getting too close, yet the more we understand ourselves, the less the likelihood of anticipating negative experiences. Developing a positive self-image is one way to gain the confidence that's needed to make new friends. The results can be surprisingly favorable.

Spiritual Values

Spiritual values are a distinct factor in moving toward a more balanced mental and physical well-being. Many people have a belief in a supreme power, some sort of God. Prayer and the power of prayer help them to keep going. The following are insights felt by some of my respondents: "God gave me the strength and courage to carry on." "Something God-given keeps me going—something inside me."

An eighty-six-year-old woman said, "I feel like I am needed."

"To be contented is the greatest thing in the world. Too much emphasis is placed on money as the only way to derive pleasure out of life. I've spent an awful lot of time with the Lord; I know that I'm never alone. I know that he protects me from wretchedness and loneliness. My faculties—I have them all. I see to read and write, usually without glasses." This lovely soul, Louise, is eighty-six years young.

Gladys referred to incidents in her early life, such as winning prizes in school and praying a lot, which gave her the faith to get through her whole life. "I don't go to church, but I have so much faith." She feels, at age seventy-eight, that one's attitude helps a person adjust to the older years.

Nellie said, "Mentally, people give up, and I will never give up. Lots of elderly people just give up reading, yet it's such a wonderful thing. But religion has helped too. I've always had a strong religious belief." She said that, mentally, she doesn't feel her eighty years.

"I have never given a thought to why I have lived to my present age," remarked Charlotte, a venerable lady of ninety-one. When I asked her what she thought might be some contributing factors, she replied, "I never stayed up all night like some people do. I tried to live a good life." She explained that religion has always been a part of her life, too.

Hope and faith provide the motivation needed to develop new interests and to remain active. Faith can be a positive contribution to help mitigate loneliness. Faith is anything believed. Faith reflects optimism. Faith in oneself is believing in oneself. Faith frequently can be a system of religious beliefs or convictions. Faith can be a confidence, a trust in a person. When we can say, "You restored my faith," we are saying a lot. Faith can involve supporting or adopting a cause or ideal. It is truly a broad concept.

There are times we speak of having faith in the outcome of something, such as faith in success. Developing faith is a means of developing our inner strength. We are expressing much when we are able to say that we have faith in a number of people in terms of their goodness, sincerity, responsibility, kindness, and principles.

Developing Closeness

An outgoing woman states, "I've always been used to a crowd around me. I've always had a family. I keep going by being close to my married daughter and her family." She feels stimulated by having the family in her life. Her relationships give her an enthusiasm for life which makes her strive for continued good health and a long life.

When I asked Evelyn, a seventy-year-old woman, what keeps her going she replied, "I'm afraid to die. I keep going for this reason. I hate to die." She paused and then continued, "I want to enjoy life. I have the means to enjoy life; therefore, I do. I love to travel. I love people, generally. I feel I have something to offer them because of my giving nature. Also, I have a lovely family, and I get a tremendous amount of love from them." At this point she revealed that she had two children, five grandchildren and three adopted grandchildren. Concluding, Evelyn said, "I have wonderful friends and have a lasting relationship with them."

The kindnesses of others keep a considerable number of our older citizens going. One remarked that she is deeply touched when treated kindly. "The older you get, the more you want someone who cares."

A typical remark made by seniors in reference to their grandchildren and great-grandchildren is, "I keep young with them." In a news article, Dr. Richard Douglas of the University of Michigan Institute of Gerontology, states:

> Socializing with other age groups keeps older people in touch with what's happening, gives them faith in the future, and helps keep them future-oriented. An especially important bond is the grandparent-grandchild relationship. Many other happy older persons unofficially adopt children from their neighborhoods or through volunteer programs.

The fact that many people, when they were young, received considerable help from their grandparents' advice and example is often overlooked. One woman (now a grandparent herself) commented on how the emotional support she received from her grandparents contributed to her adjustments to everyday living. Grandparents have played some kind of role in the early lives of many of our seniors even if not often verbalized.

Communication

The actress Joan Collins says, "Giving vent to your feelings is very healthy." Without avenues of communication we can become exceedingly lonely. Communication is essential in regard to feeling wanted, to feeling that someone cares. Communication helps to vitalize one's hopes and lends encouragement to one's life.

As I pointed out earlier, I consider communication to be a most important factor in our lives. Efforts to foster human understanding begin with communication. Much can be accomplished by sharing concerns in various settings. We stimulate thought by communicating—by conversation, exchanging ideas, translation, painting, drawing, and writing. In my own life, communication aids in eliminating feelings of insecurity. It can do the same for you.

Once I met an older couple who were deaf mutes. Their condition had existed since childhood. The wife explained in writing that they had raised six children. She had been able to make herself understood in writing, but this required much effort. While the wife did the writing in my presence, her spouse used hand signs. Their children had also learned sign language. I came away feeling a deep respect for this couple; I was greatly impressed by the depth of their communication. How tenacious they must have been through the years! Imagine the adjustments they have had to make with their children and vice versa!

Correspondence with a loved one who is not in close physical proximity can be a morale booster. This can be done in the form of writing and/or speaking. Oral communication can be done by telephone or via tape recording. An older person, alone, finds this kind of communication a vital need. This is particularly so when there are limitations in the older person's ability to reach out or reply. A daughter I know much enhanced her mother's life over the years by her steady correspondence from hundreds of miles away.

Family ties are but one avenue of communication. Senior adults attending multi-purpose centers also develop very supportive relationships. The camaraderie and the exchange of thoughts and ideas stimulates them. Readily-made friendships contribute to their overall well-being. Interaction with others increases their ability to withstand stress. The gains are more than may be obvious. Today, most senior center programs include counseling sessions. Being a participant, I have seen for myself the far-reaching benefits.

Reaching Out

Reaching out shows we care for others. Reaching out is a way of giving something of oneself. Such people tend to grow. Yet, this growth continues only with persistence. Frank H. Nelson was known for reaching out throughout his life. I first met him in 1969, and we developed a warm friendship.

Frank had been a minister in the past and, in his retirement years, served as a consultant for two senior information and referral offices under the Los Angeles County Department of Senior Citizen Affairs. He helped many older people with their problems.

In another phase of his life, Frank started a column called "Paging the Aging" in senior newspapers published in various parts of the nation. He would address problems facing seniors on a national scale as well as serve as a legislative advocate for senior adults. He was steadfast in dealing with their problems. He would often refute stereotypes which were frequently ascribed to older people. Frank

Nelson was once a representative to the White House Conference on Aging, which meets every decade.

Frank recently passed away at the age of eighty-nine. His passing was a great loss to many, including me, yet his life will always be remembered as well-spent in efforts to improve the lot of our older Americans.

Many of my contacts told me they want to be *useful*. Ed, seventy-eight, spent the first twenty-one years of his life in an orphanage and had to go to work at thirteen. He reflected, "I don't get disgusted with myself as other people do. I enjoy life, giving things away, doing for other people. It gives me a lift." He added, "You are about to absorb something from everybody with whom you come in contact. You cannot live to yourself. You have to give to others—besides getting something, you have got to give something."

Raymond, age ninety-three, said, "I love people and they bounce back at me. I love my fellowman. In my younger days I was a fraternalist."

"We should get out and meet people," said a ninety-year-old. He supplemented this by saying he still enjoys making new friends.

Anne, past seventy and single, stated that she serves as the leader with some of her friends; she takes the initiative. Of her earlier life, in relation to friends, she said, "I kept growing. They didn't grow the way I did. I appreciate certain people more than I did in the past." As to her relatives: "I have a different lifestyle than they have. We don't have much in common." In our conversation, I found this person to be helpful in others' lives. Her activities reflect this. "Inwardly I am a happy person," she concluded.

Gordon, a man in his sixties serving as a moderator in a senior discussion group feels that people keep him going. He said, "I have an incredible feeling when talking with people and listening to what they have to say. We have mutually discovered the depths and vistas of each other—a never-ending source of amazement." Another senior made this observation: "When you suffer loss, you appreciate what is still there."

Feelings of Insecurity

Older people constantly undergo changes, some more pronounced than others. Feelings of insecurity can assail seniors even when they have previously had motivation and hope for the future. Their spirit fluctuates over a period of time, more so when getting up in years.

I had a conversation with Nora, eighty-two, someone whom I had spoken with more than a year earlier. Once again I asked, "What keeps you going?" Previously she had stated that many kinds of activities were part of her daily living, but now she wanted me to understand things were different. "Life is like tissue paper. It doesn't keep together a long time, but that is what keeps me going." Nora said that her physical stamina had declined and this had made her feel insecure and less productive. She was also having trouble in her relationship with her second husband, an eighty-six-year-old man she had married fourteen years earlier.

I know Nora well. She is tenacious in getting things done, in spite of her frailties. She is able to get about reasonably well and continues in her healthy pursuits: keeping up her small apartment, visiting friends and relatives away from her area, pursuing an active interest in the daily news, and being friendly to those in her housing complex. Her feelings of insecurity are a mixture of depression and doubts about her ability to carry on vivaciously. I felt that Nora, active her entire life, now needed a certain continued recognition and warmth that her husband wasn't readily showing her. Her visits with friends and relatives away from her area, including her husband's, was a meaningful way to improve the quality of her life.

Grief and Family Attitudes

The death of a mate can be a crucial loss in a person's life. How can we deal with such overwhelming grief? People in such circumstances seek ways and means to alleviate their sorrow. Some tend to snap back by becoming involved in outside interests. Others make an effort to reach out to others.

In losing a lifetime partner, a person must take on *many responsibilities never held before.* Learning to handle their lives without assistance is a large adjustment. It is essential to plan ahead. The widow and widower must learn that they possess more abilities than they thought they had. Inner strengths emerge that did not previously show themselves. The fact that they are now forced to depend on themselves bring these strengths forward. A renewed outlook on life may result; self-esteem often increases. Sometimes the gains are made easier with the help of counseling. As referred to before, most senior centers are equipped with this service.

Widows, in some instances, may have a family to turn to, either theirs or their deceased spouse's family. A widow must remember that she still is part of a family and is not really alone. One woman, in referring to her deceased spouse's family, had this to say: "I feel they are my family; they still belong. It's important that you have had a good relationship and then it will still continue."

Loneliness

Loneliness can be devastating. People can be terribly lonely even if they are not in nursing homes, which is typically a place where people feel lonesome. Even with average health and the ability to fend for themselves, some seniors have limited interests and faith. They have nothing to insulate them from loneliness. I am referring to those who do not bounce back from loss and cannot easily offset loneliness.

Losing her spouse the year before, Katherine, an eighty-four-year-old, said, "Until it happens, you don't know how it feels to be alone." She wasn't able to overcome her feelings of loneliness because she lacked interests as well as faith in her ability to adopt any. If we become withdrawn, living a sheltered life and allowing isolation to set in, we lose self-reliance and self-confidence.

Off-Setting Loneliness

Close family ties can distinctly improve a person's ability to make adjustments. Living with someone also enhances this ability. Feeling that we are loved, that we have someone to reach out to us, is essential. Improved social outlets result in physical gains as well as emotional ones.

A mother in her eighties living alone said: "It's the sharing, getting together with the family. It is not only *having* family, but it's the *sharing*. The *closeness* is what counts."

To develop these social outlets, we need an improved image of ourselves. What can be done to obtain the improved image? Here I find that Senior Peer Counseling is helpful. In this setting, people gain confidence by expressing themselves. A more positive attitude emerges. Senior Peer Counseling, for example, is located in senior centers and hospital medical centers, and frequently offered for free or, at the most, a nominal charge.

What else helps the self-image? We have touched on the benefits of volunteer work. Nearby hospitals can provide this form of activity; one can be a companion to shut-ins. Also, senior centers use volunteers in many settings. People make friends by attending nutrition programs in these centers. The luncheon is at a nominal cost and usually held five days per week. One's self-image can also improve through various senior center activities and classes. And, occasionally, a romance develops in these centers.

Claire, over seventy, likes to communicate with people. She said, "If you have no one, and no one to look forward to, you just drift." Also, she enjoys reminiscing. She also likes savoring the past—referring to the wonderful times she had in her younger days. Occasionally the past, or savoring the past, can be over-emphasized. More emphasis should be placed on present-day activities. As Claire stated, she likes communicating with people; this human contact should keep her from dwelling too much on the past.

The late Simone de Beauvoir, the French writer, in *The Coming of Age,* describes the characteristics of the famous painter, Monet:

> He was endowed with a surprising capacity for work; he had very good health; he was surrounded with affection; he loved life; and this was how he painted himself, in what might be called the exuberance of old age—upright, merry, with a fine clear complexion, an abundant beard, his eyes full of life and gaiety.

I would like to draw attention to the point de Beauvoir makes that Monet was "surrounded with affection." This is a major accomplishment in a person's life. What good fortune *affection* can be! I'll elaborate on this concept shortly. First, I would like to discuss the phenomena of touching.

Touching

In forming relationships and developing affections, a seemingly inconsequential matter is the gesture of *touch.* What value does touching really have? How frequently has a firm handshake left an indelible impression? As I related earlier, my father and I were separated for some years when I was a child. As a late teenager, I was reunited with him. A reasonably good friendship developed. Later, when he was in his eighties, he contracted pneumonia.

On a particular visit to the hospital, my father in bed appeared heavily sedated. His eyes were closed. I gently took hold of the fingers of one of his hands. I called out to him. He slowly opened his eyes, squeezing my fingers in a certain firmness of acknowledgement. For several minutes his eyes remained fixed upon me with our fingers clasped together. He was unable to express himself, yet we seemed to have a depth of understanding. It remains an experience that I will forever remember. In life I was destined never to see him again after that day.

There is much to be said for braille reading and sign language among the deaf. The hands are important in this support system. Among families where deafness may be prevalent, touch and sign are significant means to communicate. The many braille institutes throughout the world should be commended for the manner in which they benefit people with these handicaps. Recently, I read an absorbing book: *In Silence: Growing Up Hearing in a Deaf World* by Ruth Sidransky, which brings to light the experiences of deaf people.

Recently, the TV station KCET presented a documentary film on the tactile phenomenon, or touch. The film first included animals, and then people. In a controlled experiment monkeys in need of physical contact were shown. A long period without physical contact can result in emotional trauma. It was also revealed that denying touch for an extended period can cause brain damage, as reflected among a monkey colony.

The film went on to examine the value of touch therapy among boys and girls who suffer from anxiety and depression. The children were given animals to keep as pets, and the conclusion was drawn that pet ownership can have a strong effect on survival. We can calm ourselves by touching animals, bringing a kind of peace and tranquility. Having a dog or cat is a good way to offset loneliness. Birds can also be beneficial in this way. Pet ownership has many benefits that promote well-being and better morale. This can make living alone far less lonely.

Touch aids in building social and emotional relationships among couples of all ages. Touching can improve closeness. Would older adults withdraw from a friend lovingly placing an arm around them? Probably not. We have all seen how an embrace can quiet a child.

I recently came across a book on touching that I highly recommend. It is by Helen Colton, entitled *The Gift of Touch*. She broadly amplifies the timeliness of this subject.

Love and Affection

The concept of touch includes other considerations, such as showing care and a certain degree of affection. The ability to reach out is a most valuable trait. It can be accomplished in a variety of ways, such as initiating a phone call or a conversation with a neighbor or friend. However, when it is accomplished, concern and affection will enhance any relationship.

Affection and love intertwine. To keep going, to add to our years, and to have a confident outlook, the concept of love must be brought into focus.

Love is multifaceted. Below the surface there is much love in most people. It shows up in many different ways.

For example, I saw love surface in the audience during the film *E.T.* The audience projected care toward an extraterrestrial creature.

It is reasonable to say that outward love, as a rule, is not sufficiently expressed among most humans. This is true of people of all ages. Why can't we be as spontaneous as children in showing love?

In cultivating relationships with family and friends we must give prominence to love. We are born with a need for love in the same way we are born needing to be touched. Throughout life, the issue of love will exist. As well-attested, the need for love is not lessened because we grow older. In an article entitled, "Affection—Especially at Age 75" (August 3, 1980, *Los Angeles Times*) Jim Sanderson makes the point that:

> Every human being requires conversation and friendship, but why do we assume that the needs of older people stop there? The body may creak a little, but there is not arteriosclerosis of the emotions. (Copyright, 1980, Los Angeles Times. Reprinted by permission.)

Love gives added dimension to whatever fulfillment we find in life. Giving and receiving love can be more motivating than almost anything else. It doesn't come easily to everyone, but we can all get in touch with ourselves and learn to love who we are, a relevant touchstone in developing love for others.

Whatever love may mean to seniors, it is a strong motivator. There are many interpretations of its meaning because there are many different kinds of love. A few basic ones are physical, emotional, and spiritual love.

Excellent statements dealing with love can be found in *Real Love, What It Is and How to Find It* by Theodore Isaac Rubin, M.D.:

> The stronger our sense of self, knowing who we are, how we feel, being in touch with our priorities in life, our values, (what is and isn't important to us), and our goals, interests and desires, the better equipped we are for loving.

Later in his book, Dr. Rubin expresses:

> Making peace with the aging process increases love of self, love of the life process, and enhances aliveness and feelings of love generally.

A close male friend of mine, an octogenarian, speaks of autumn love. I like the implication of this kind of love. Among older adults, the attractions can be somewhat different in autumn love. The spiritual values can be deeper. Physical attraction has a certain degree of meaning, but at the same time the quietness of the mind generates a depth of feeling. Common interests and common experiences usually enter into the love relationship. There is a mutuality that rests on a strong foundation.

Romance and Sexuality

Couples want to enjoy romance to the utmost. Maturity has its compensations. The couples are usually more settled with leanings toward deep sincerity, commitment, trust, and respect. In many instances, expectations are reduced because people at this age are likely to have reached some sort of status quo. More attention can therefore be given to the relationship. This allows the two participants to grow even closer, because in autumn love, there is often a compelling concern between the loved ones to consummate deeper feelings as never before. Being less inhibited, such individuals are less afraid to show love.

In *Sexuality and Aging,* edited by Robert L. Solnick, Ruth B. Weg, in her chapter "The Physiology of Sexuality in Aging," states:

> Evidence is overwhelming that the need for intimate, affective relationships exists for most men and women all through life. . . . In a climate of awareness and concern for human needs and wants, we shall see an important move away from the goal-oriented passion of youth to the person-oriented intimacy of the mature and later years.

In this same book, Margaret Neiswender Reedy, in a chapter, "What Happens to Love," says:

> What is most valued between married lovers in later life? When we looked at the way older men and women described their relationships, we found that, as a group, older lovers valued emotional security most in their love relationships. . . . Respect was rated the second most important aspect of love for older lovers. . . . Respect for some older couples means being able to be good friends as well as lovers.

In the book *Sexuality in the Later Years,* edited by Ruth B. Weg, Nan Corly and Judy Maes Zarit, in the chapter "Old and Alone: The Unmarried in Later Life," state:

By focusing too much on the achievement of orgasm, we may interfere with these other equally valid expressions of sexuality and closeness (i.e., caressing, touching, feelings of warmth and closeness, and sexual interest in general), in a special type of intimate relationship.

At another point they indicate:

A relaxation of personal and social attitudes might benefit single older women and help them to accept their sexuality—or at least to experience it—as fully as some men seem to accept and experience theirs.

Gordon S. Walbroehl, M.D., in the article "Educating Elderly Patients About Sex," in *Geriatric Consultant* (May/June 1990) adds to this discussion of love and sexuality:

Sexuality, you can assure your elderly patients, is a basic instinct that is retained relatively late in patients with even the most devastating disease. Patients with Alzheimer's disease, for instance, have been reported to be sexually active with their partners, yet not remember their own name.... Sexual expression, we all know, changes as one ages. But it does not automatically end at a given point. As Vanderbilt Manley points out, sexual activity can even improve for couples who have been together for many years. "There's much less emphasis on performance, and much more on just the joy and pleasure and totality of sex," she says. (Reprinted by permission of Gordon S. Walbroehl, M.D.)

Andrew M. Greeley, in his book, *Faithful Attractions: Discovering Intimacy, Love and Fidelity in American Marriage* (1991), discusses "the surprising truths revealed by the provocative new national Gallup survey." A questionnaire was given to couples of several age groups. The following is from the chapter, "Sex Over Sixty":

> It is simply not true that after a certain age in life the importance of the sexual bond diminishes. Those over sixty think it more important than do younger people. They may not engage in it as often, but it does not follow that they think it has lost its importance. . . . Those over sixty are no less likely than those under sixty to say their spouse is attractive and 55% say their spouse is a skilled lover (46% for those under sixty). . . .

Dostoevski, the prolific Russian writer, writing on the theme of love said, "Love will teach us all things. . . ." If we pause and reflect a moment, this simple observation can stir our minds, as we can interpret it in various ways. In allowing love to enter into our lives, we give an added dimension to our existence.

A number of seniors have confirmed that love relationships help keep them going. People's views of marriage in the later years vary. Companionship often brings deeper feelings than ever before.

On a TV program called "Love Connection," a ninety-year-old man, out of three possible choices, picked an eighty-four-year-old woman for a date. They developed a nice friendship, planning another date together. The man was three times a widower, yet was a spunky person with a good sense of humor and in good physical shape. Both admired, complimented, and were physically attracted to each other. Watching the chemistry between these two older adults was enjoyable.

One gentleman said that he added years to his life because he remarried at sixty-nine. My readers will probably agree that remarrying offers many advantages. The reasons remarrying adds years to one's life varies with each person. In the case of the sixty-nine-year-old, we might conclude he found fulfillment by remarrying—having a companion instead of remaining alone.

A live-in relationship can also offer stability. Sharing feelings and developing a commitment can add to the relationship. With many, loneliness and isolation are reasons for seeking companionship. When in a lonely state and feeling down, a person often feels out of step with the universe. How many are complete within themselves, or really want to remain alone?

An eighty-four-year-old man raised that very question in a discussion: How many people are complete within themselves? He made the point that basically every human being needs another person in their life, and that there is a need for communication at various times. To be connected with other people is a way to improve the quality of life. Is it any wonder that developing a close relationship can add to a person's adjustments?

With older adults, the sex factor cannot be minimized. Fantasies about sex exist at all ages, and some preoccupation with the desire to have a loved one is prominent among single seniors. In addition to sexual interests, both men and women can enjoy being in one another's company, developing attachments, and sharing commitment.

Different Forms of Love

In *Add Life to Your Years,* Dr. Frank S. Caprio describes the meaning of love:

What is love?
Love is living, love is giving, love is warmth.
Love is courage, love is wisdom, love is understanding.
Love is forgiveness, love is kindness. Love is protection, security, belonging. Love is creative self-expression.
Love is the sharing of laughter.
Love is emotional and sexual maturity. Love is building. Love is life's fulfillment. . . .

Dr. Caprio's comprehensive definition of love would seem to hold something for everyone. Further, is it possible to feel and to share so many kinds of love? Why not? What do we have to lose? Our immediate world may improve, may open up. We can plant the idea in our minds that *love need not fade.*

Quoted in part, "Love," by Roy Croft, from the book *Best Loved Poems of the American People,* illustrates the mutual benefits of a love relationship:

I love you,
Not only for what you are,
But for what I am
When I am with you.

I love you,
Not only for what
You have made of yourself,
But for what
You are making of me.

    These short lines express the sharing and growth that are the results of a love relationship. This poem can make us reflect and appreciate someone we care about. The awareness of how much love can mean touches the soul—if we are lucky we have understood this through a relationship in our own life. If not, we have most certainly observed it in someone we've known.

    I once met a man who was in charge of a newsstand. He was wearing an attractive gold pendant on a chain. It caught my attention. It was the size of a half-dollar broken in half with rough edges. It had some kind of inscription. When I asked what it meant, he answered that the inscription was in Hebrew and that his wife wears the other half. He added that he had been happily married to her for fifty-one years. His happiness, in turn, made me feel happy.

    We can say that *love is life.* If we miss love, we also miss life. Plainly, the value of love in anyone's life cannot be underestimated; *love makes life meaningful.* When a TV sports program interviewed a seventy-six-year-old harness horse racer, he said resolutely, "If there is something you love, you live longer."

    Even when we lose someone we love, a part of the love remains. We have the memories of the special times with them. We cherish what they added to our lives, and we learn to carry on with their warmth and spirit.

When I asked a woman past sixty-five what kept her going, she replied: "I love life. I love nature. I enjoy my family. I let them live their own lives. I have many interests, and I have an open mind. I feel that I learn something new every day because I love life. I like people and I talk to them. I enjoy physical and mental activity. Am I unusual? I don't think I am. I am growing older gracefully. I am happy from within. You must be happy yourself before you can make someone else happy."

When we say we *love life,* we are saying much. When we love life, we keep an open mind, keep learning, and share what we find. There are many ways to develop the ability to love, but they all stem from knowing who we are and what will make us happy.

Developing a warmth for people, relationships, and an interest in various activities assists in our overall well-being. Being deeply involved in an activity often means one loves it. Some years ago, Smiley Blanton, the writer and psychiatrist, in *Love or Perish,* made this observation:

> Another remarkable example of what love can do for the human spirit was afforded by the French painter, Renoir. That modern master worked joyously at his beloved easel even though he was so crippled by rheumatism during his last two decades that he had to be carried everywhere in a chair and could not hold the paint brushes in his fingers. He would have the brushes tied to his wrist, and in this manner produced some of his most beautiful work in the years before his death at the age of seventy-eight. The power of love to triumph over all adversity perhaps never received more awe-inspiring expression than when this heroic old

man remarked to his friends that he had no right to complain, since "things might have been worse."

Life Satisfactions

Some of us are more fortunate than others in matters of love. Some are blessed with a variety of rich and meaningful relationships without much effort. And there are others who take for granted the love they are given. Emotional support should not be taken lightly, yet now and then we will do this with our loved ones. It is vital to be thoughtful. Giving should be our main concern. We should pause a moment to think what it would be like to be alone without our loved ones. *People need each other.*

A person who radiated love and compassion and was vitally interested in our older Americans inspired the University of Southern California to dedicate a building in her honor—The Ethel Percy Andrus Gerontology Center. The 30 million-plus members of the American Association for Retired Persons (AARP) is a great testimony to Ethel Andrus. Miss Andrus was a staunch pioneer in the gerontology field. Here is one of her thoughtful statements from her *Power of Years:*

> Do we not know persons who progress through life solving their own problems, living purposefully, lending a helping hand to others where needed and keeping love in their hearts for their fellow man? These persons have developed an inner beauty that does much to soften wrinkles and sagging chins, to lessen irregularities of features and even to challenge chronological age itself.

Like Ethel Percy Andrus, many people are able to *radiate* tenderness.

When we are in touch with our feelings, we can become more in touch with the people around us. We can contribute to others. The end result is that we are more in touch with life itself. As one widow put it, "Everybody should laugh a little, sing a little, and love a little—simply because they're alive."

This reminds me of an anecdote my friends relayed to me. At a dance where various age groups were gathered, my friends became acquainted with a man and his wife. The man looked so very proper, dressed well, and had a little mustache. He volunteered the information that he was ninety-two years of age—his *fifth* wife being eighty-one. He added that he does no boozing, no drinking, and has "been into clean living." Then, with emphasis, he raised his arms in a spirit of drama and remarked, "But romance! Romance!"

Chapter VI
Personal Values

> Every time a value is born, existence takes on a new meaning; every time one dies, some part of that meaning passes away.
> —Joseph Wood Krutch
> *"Love*—or the Life and Death of a Value," *The Modern Temper*

The significance of personal values is frequently overlooked. When people speak of "values," they are generally referring to social values, those dealing with our cultural or social institutions. Yet the personal inner values of mature adults are frequently vital and, as such, are a distinct factor in understanding what keeps older citizens going.

There has been a tendency in our culture to believe that we are living in an age where values have deteriorated. However, there are many who disagree with this viewpoint and who themselves demonstrate a fierce loyalty to specific convictions and beliefs. Many older adults fit into this category. They possess a certain vigor, a spirit of belief and faith that is the result of having developed deep personal values over many years. Such treasured values are multi faceted and, when incorporated into one's way of life, can provide sustenance and direction. Values benefit people of all age groups and, fortunately, the values of many of our seniors are passed on to their children and succeeding generations.

Personal and social values overlap to some extent. As Clarence Marsh Case, in his *Essays on Social Values,* commented, "Personal values are primarily, even uniquely, individual selections, but they are socially conditioned in their origin."

Vern Bengtson, a professor of sociology in the field of geriatrics, lists the following social values: achievement, freedom, service to mankind, equality, friendship, loyalty to your own (family), patriotism, financial comfort, respect, possessions, and experience.

Social values have deep significance in any culture, but personal convictions are what lend individuals the most support. They must be cultivated by one's experience. Harold H. Titus, in his *Living Issues in Philosophy,* points out:

> From the time of the ancient Greeks to the present, many philosophers have stressed three values as superior to all others: goodness, beauty, and truth. These values are said to be self-sufficient. . . . To goodness, beauty and truth some would add happiness. Others would subsume these values under the heading of religious value.

The Manner in Which Values Take Hold

Early values are usually carried into later life. Our early years form our basic outlooks in a variety of ways: family living, schools, peers, mass communication or media, to name a few. These early beliefs become part of our overall value system, guiding us and affecting our attitudes and decisions. Raths, Harmin, and Simon, in *Values and Teaching: Working with Values in the Classroom,* state:

> The development of values is a personal and life-long process. It is not something that is completed by early adulthood.... one of the criteria for a value is that it is something that penetrates a person's life, that it uses some of a person's limited energy and resources, that it really counts in behavioral decisions.

Simon, Howe, and Kirschenbaum, in *Values Clarification,* assert, "Value indicators are often forged from actions, attitudes, aspirations, beliefs, convictions, interests, likes, dislikes, goals, and purposes."

Cultivating our values not only produces inner *stability,* but also *productivity.* Some personal values help determine how other values will develop in our growing years and throughout our lifetime. There is little doubt that the values we develop are colored by what we have been brought up to believe, such as traditional values of freedom, individuality, love, and hope.

Harold H. Titus, in *Living Issues in Philosophy,* quotes Abraham H. Maslow, who pointed to certain basic values:

> ... the human being is so constructed that he presses toward fuller and fuller being and this means pressing toward what most people would call good values, toward serenity, kindness, courage, knowledge, honesty, love, unselfishness, and goodness.

The significance of Maslow's statement might vary at different ages. Some of the values he mentions are commonly held by older people.

I have compiled a list of personal values in addition to those mentioned by Maslow. This list comes from a variety of sources. Although I have tried to supply a strong sample, I've made no attempt to make this list all-inclusive:

creativity	imagination
contentment	faith
self-appreciation	inquisitiveness
sociability	perseverance
action	a sense of purpose
patience	a constitutional determi-
security	nation or fortitude
spirituality	independence
self-discovery	standing on ideals and
tolerance	principles
adjusting to change	equality
friendship	good deeds
responsibility	compassion
determination	education
leisure	cleanliness
folk wisdom	hope
cooperation	adventure
tenderness	meditation
joy	dignity
integrity	vitality
cheerfulness	youthfulness
humanness	a sense of humor
goals	adaptability
self-control	

Does this list pose any new values you would like to take on? Can we say that this list of values and those referred to by other writers can fit into a retirement setting? I believe they can. This group of values reflect many I've embraced over the years. I have given serious thought to those values which have given me a stronger sense of self-confidence.

Recently, I had the opportunity to present a similar list to a men's group at a senior center (of the thirty men, most were past sixty-five). I wrote a list of values on a blackboard and suggested the group members pick out three that applied in their present-day living and for which they had deep convictions. At least six of the men indicated that they would pick them all. The choices were*:

knowledge	8	compassion	3
friendship	7	truth	2
tolerance	5	serenity	2
responsibility	4	unselfishness	2
beauty	3	education	2
kindness	3	inquisitiveness	2
honesty	3		

*Eleven values not shown were given one choice each.

These men appear to place much importance on knowledge, which seems to be fundamental to these men. It is understandable that friendship and tolerance are high on the list as well. These seniors meet once a week and find this group a valuable medium through which they can express themselves, learn, and find comradeship.

Changing Values at Retirement Age

At retirement, new personal values emerge. From a work setting to a leisure-time setting, patterns of living change, often causing certain values to be discarded and others to become important. It is a good idea to check the values that currently concern us. They can further one's motivation in day-to-day living. Sometimes we gain insight from a new value. Such an acquisition can come about unexpectedly, perhaps by becoming involved in a learning activity with others.

We might lend more excitement to our lives by searching out a value that has long been taken for granted. A new spark might be generated, or interest in a discarded value may be renewed. A monograph prepared by the School of Social Work at Syracuse University reads:

> Old age may be a time of decreasing physical activity, but it may also serve as a time for evaluating one's life, a time of sharing experiences, a time to help others, a time to defend certain prized values. (Reprinted by permission.)

Relevant here is a life sketch of another senior, Jim. At the end of this sketch, I will list what I see as values he has had earlier in life combined with the values he currently holds.

Jim: The Varied Influences and the Coping Mechanisms in His Life

Jim is a senior with whom I have developed a warm friendship in recent years. He is currently seventy-five, unmarried, and is a warm and modest human being to whom one can easily relate.

His weathered features mark his years in deep lines across his forehead and down his cheeks. His eyes peer out intensely, looking squarely at you. A neatly trimmed white mustache and a full head of wavy gray hair add a distinctiveness to his appearance. His clothing has a western flavor that reflects outdoor living. Jim has a polite and gentle manner. You feel that he is absorbing every word you say.

Our discussion began when I referred to the adversity in peoples' lives. Jim immediately responded, "Negative forces have aided me, made me stand up against the elements." Jim gave the analogy of tree during a storm. "They are able to bend a little, which is what keeps them from breaking." Jim stretched his arms out wide and said, "I possess great curiosity—ZING! Others weaken and fold up like a delicate flower. You've got to have resilience in life. I don't let problems stop me from getting what I want."

Let us turn back the clock in this friend's life. After the age of six, Jim had a stepfather. "He gave me love, his way, without affection. He was a perfectionist. I just couldn't please him. My stepfather wanted to teach me my ABC's. He came on strong. He wanted everything to be in order. He was meticulous. I had to have high ideals and standards." Jim paused and then said, "He did the best he could, but didn't understand my feelings. He wanted me to follow in his footsteps. His vision was limited.

"My stepfather sometimes hurt me," said Jim. "He did play sports with me; we had games together, but he had to win." Jim cited an incident that occurred when he was eight while playing croquet. "I had tears in my eyes when I lost, but I knew I could never beat him," Jim solemnly stated. "His sense of humor was bad. I had some hate for him. I sometimes wanted to run away."

There wasn't much agreement between his parents. "My mother was loosely put together. She was always searching for some kind of happiness, such as beauty. She seemed to need recognition, lots of attention, and constant love." I asked Jim what he meant by his mother being "loosely put together." He replied, "She wasn't too rigid, never liked to put on airs, and wasn't worried what people thought of her. She had her problems, but basically she was direct, sincere, and honest, with high morals." Jim said he had a lot of feeling for his mother and her problems. At age fifteen, when his parents had marital difficulties, he tried to counsel them. Jim feels that he played an important role as sort of counselor, adding, "It gave me self-assurance and pleasure to help get them together. I was building some sort of self-esteem."

His stepfather divorced his mother when Jim was still young. His mother had a nervous breakdown, but eventually improved, becoming fairly stable after a time. Jim said that she was not much of a force in his younger life. He favored his grandmother over his mother. "My grandmother gave me unconditional love—she was very understanding." He declared that "if I didn't have a belief in myself, I would not have been able to stand my stepfather."

Jim did not complete high school. "I wouldn't study. I wanted to be out with nature. I had an overabundance of curiosity about nature, but lacked the patience to study. The only subject I liked in school was geography."

At twenty-one, before the Great Depression began, Jim went into the military. "I was a patriotic kid. Both my grandfathers were Civil War veterans." He spoke of having a hard time in the service. "I hated authority." He admits that it was a good experience because he was able to work and be provided for at a time when few outside jobs were available.

After a three-year hitch, Jim reenlisted for another two years. "I had a guilt complex about not having completed high school when I reentered the army. I wanted to be a pilot but I had to brush up on math. I was not sure I could make it. It was a blind spot. I built a wall." Jim explained that he had failed math in high school and had allowed his failure to carry on. "Then I let it go—I gave up. It was bad for my morale. I made a hell of a big mistake. Still, overall, I had faith in myself. I left the army. I found a woman who gave me inspiration and I married her."

I asked Jim how his wife had inspired him. Jim replied, "She could see possibilities in me. She was real. She believed in me and helped to change my life around. We had a lot in common." A pattern developed where Jim and his wife would read books together dealing with philosophy and psychology. "I had an exposure to growth," he said.

Developing an expertise with his hands, Jim became skilled in auto and truck welding, eventually owning his own shop. He acquired other skills—carpentry, electricity, plumbing—and did much to renovate his own home.

Jim has come a long way over the years, and he is still growing. Once, more than thirty years ago, when he felt that there was something missing in his life, he learned how to meditate. "It's getting away from the past, living in the *now*. It makes you aware of something greater than yourself, something in life and nature, tranquil, quiet and peaceful. It calms the mind. It's a daily thing and helps my center," expressed Jim enthusiastically. "I use meditation to regulate my emotions. It's been an asset in helping me to find myself. I'm still looking."

Today, as a senior adult, he is busy and happy. In his current activities, he is a volunteer in the DOVES Program (Dedicated Older Volunteers in Educational Services), assisting children in remedial instruction in public schools. He is also an ombudsman, volunteering his services in nursing homes to older patients whose difficulties in making adjustments require him to listen and talk to patients as well as administrative representatives.

In addition to these activities, Jim likes to read, especially self-improvement and motivational books. He has been active in senior support groups where people share feelings and ideas. At one point he emphasized, "I want to see the world *better—at peace.*"

I could give many illustrations of how Jim continues to grow and work toward becoming a more complete human being. Change can be initiated—at any age—as Jim proved when he said, "I have come further in the last six years than in all the rest of my years put together. For me, life is like a jigsaw puzzle—in the end the pieces are coming together."

Jim's Personal Values

From Maslow's List:
   serenity
   kindness
   courage
   knowledge
   honesty
   love

My Own Estimation:
   sociability
   self-discovery
   imagination
   faith
   inquisitiveness
   a sense of purpose
   hope
   meditation

Jim's Social Values

patriotism   responsibility
family loyalty   volunteering
compassion   adaptability
resilience

There is no doubt that those of you reading might see the things which have influenced Jim's life could have also influenced your own. It might be fascinating to compare your own values to Jim's.

Respondents' Values

I should note that when I asked my respondents what kept them going and what they felt was responsible for their long life, their unprompted replies often pointed to personal values. At first, I made no deliberate attempt to discuss values with them. Later on, during some interviews, values were touched on. I was greatly impressed with the impact values had on people. The worth that people placed on carrying on was far-reaching.

Certain beliefs, ideals, values—whatever we care to call them—are prized more than others at various times in our lives. Russell, a retired widower, age seventy-two, who had been without his spouse for some time, said: "When you can't work anymore, you kind of feel guilty. You build a little nest. You live right, so you feel right. I've had paticnce—which is the reason why I've lived so long."

Martha, an outgoing and well-liked seventy-three-year-old who had raised a family, stated: "I am a person who has been able to adjust to change, to adapt to my surroundings. Life is one long learning experience. You are bound to absorb something from everybody you come into contact with.'' She amplified her philosophy: ''You can't give to yourself. You have to give to others; besides getting something, you must give something.''

At age seventy-eight, Nora, an independent and resourceful woman, remarked: ''Whatever you put into life, you get out. It is not what you *think* you are, it is *who* you *are*. It shows up in your character. You have to live it every day. You have to build a character.''

Lucy, a sprightful eighty-one-year-old who had many friends among her neighbors said, ''I live my life with happiness and youthfulness. I never think that I am old.''

Evelyn, a widow of seventy-six, reflected, ''People should look with beauty in their eyes instead of hatred.'' She added that such thinking had stimulated her in her own life. She said, ''When you find solace in the lives of others, your own life is changed.''

At age seventy-one, Kay feels that her life has been filled with satisfaction. She keeps certain standards and believes they are necessary to her happiness and contentment. She said, ''Life has been a vital, exciting experience.''

A petite ninety-year-old, Harriet, who lives in a trailer park, had a lovely sense of humor and a glow about her. She expressed these feelings: ''You should have your own philosophy. You must work for it, not carry over someone else's. I learn on 'mind over matter.' '' She confided that she leans on God. Continuing, she said, ''Growth is important.'' She studies when it is quiet, after twelve at night.

I later learned, as might be expected, that she has many friends where she lives.

Are We Prisoners of Our Past?

In Morton Puner's *Getting the Most Out of Your Fifties,* the late scientist and gerontologist, Rene Dubos, at age seventy-one, said:

> [People] should retain as long as possible, the ability to experience many kinds of situations, to discover what they like and what makes them productive and happy. They should not become prisoners of their past too early in life.

Do we necessarily have to remain prisoners of the past at any stage of life? What are we doing to produce some good for ourselves? How do we promote a feeling of happiness? We need not become prisoners of our past if we dwell on the good that we see in ourselves.

Earlier, I mentioned that values create inner *stability* and *productivity.* We might add the values of contentment and serenity to Dubos' statement "to discover what we like." Finding what makes us "productive and happy" is worth the time and trouble, as it brings a contented serenity.

Believing in Ourselves: Enlisting Certain Values

It is vital to offset negative events with convictions. In Howard Whitman's *A Brighter Later Life,* the famous dancer, Ruth St. Denis (now deceased), explained:

Creative thinking and enthusiasm for life itself cannot be accounted for. I don't know where they come from; I do know that a great many people start out in life with these attributes, but at some point lose them. The grave happenings in life cause this . . . if in this dark hour of defeat, loneliness, and misery, one does not have some basic spiritual principle—with any earthly name you want to give it—then he will never recover. He will then join the large group of people who in their last years and sometimes even earlier, are a dreary drag on their families and society.

What has supported me is the wonderful faith and belief which was taught to me as a child. I have been more or less kept alive by my beloved friends, sometimes only one of them, which gives me a tremendous foundation to build on.

Ruth St. Denis' values, creativity, enthusiasm, faith and belief, lend a spark to daily living. We cannot afford to lose these types of values which offer us support.

If we sufficiently believe in ourselves, we develop added good thoughts, simultaneously improving our personal values and ideals. To reach a higher level in this regard, we need to be selective in the thoughts we have of ourselves.

A young gerontology student attending a senior citizen discussion group expressed what *faith* can do: "People have faith in me which gives me moral support. This [in turn] gives me hope and determination."

Marian, age seventy-four, touched on faith in my discussion with her. She cupped her hands, looked at me squarely, and remarked, "When you've got *faith,* you've got the world in your hands."

I asked Katherine, eighty-six, how she fills her time. She replied, "I don't have enough time for what I've got to do." Continuing, she said that she is aided by "the holy spirit" within herself. She goes "on living day by day" just doing what is in front of her. But this doesn't mean her life is boring. Katherine mentioned having made a cross-continental bus trip by herself to visit relatives the previous summer.

A number of those interviewed voiced a need to develop the value of *understanding* life. This relates to tolerance, getting along with others, and appreciating other people's opinions as well as one's own.

Many also placed importance on growing and being able to change along with the world—"to be on your toes." The consensus was that at no time should one limit oneself. The hardships that were prevalent in their earlier lives helped those interviewed to develop a *strong intestinal fortitude*—an excellent value. Close to this are perseverance and steadfastness. These values mirror the personal values of a senior who had overcome the handicap of being unable to hear or speak. She expressed herself well to her spouse and others by sign language and writing.

A large number of older persons believed that a good carry-over in later life was a basic cheerfulness and a sense of humor. A number of my contacts placed importance on being productive and happy. Others expressed the importance of patience, hope, and faith. These older adults found it vital to have something to hang on to. Faith plays a distinctive role in their lives. With faith, they tend to generate a strong belief in themselves, as well as in the world about them.

About 18 years ago, I had the pleasure of meeting Louis Zamperini, a former Olympic track star. "You have to have goals in life," he said when I asked what kept him going. I did not have the chance to ask him to elaborate on the goals he was referring to. However, this former Olympic star contributed much in the way of character and charisma. Athletically, young people look up to those who have made a name for themselves. No doubt it was a challenge to Mr. Zamperini to help guide boys and girls as well as inspire people of all ages. In fact, at the time of our interview, Mr. Zamperini was involved in church work with young people and seniors in meetings to deal with community problems. His "goals in life" more than likely had to do with his church work as well as athletic involvements.

Vital Thoughts in Shaping One's Values

A.H. Maslow in *The Farther Reaches of Human Nature* states:

> The more man knows about his own nature, his deep wishes, his temperament, his constitution, what he seeks and yearns for, and what really satisfies him, the more effortless, automatic . . . become his value choices. This is one of the great Freudian discoveries and one which is often overlooked.

One could spend months and years improving life along these lines. These thoughts represent a challenge in the process of shaping one's values.

Understandably, when we are older and have experienced much of life, we cannot begin to initiate far-reaching insights and changes. Yet, at least we have the option to strive for Maslow's vision. We can follow through, regardless of our years, to make some of these thoughts a further reality.

Although we are constantly faced with the practical necessities of daily living, I feel that we can simultaneously search for meaning and value. There are older people who desire to become more involved, to stay active, and there are some who withdraw, leading a more leisurely and reflective kind of existence. As a result, the values of each type of individual can vary.

Effects from the Negative Side of Life

Limited self-esteem or self-worth can influence one's state of mind. Such views, for example, affect adjustments to change, contentment, faith, and a sense of purpose. Negative experiences can erase personal values. A large portion of older citizens live quite a limited existence where values are seldom referred to, yet they have values.

People who feel life is passing them by have little thought of values. Who is supposed to have values? Not those who possess very little hope. One's life has to radiate *some* hope. It is only then that values can have meaning. Take the personal value of love as an example. Many believe we must first love ourselves before we can love others and allow the value of love to have meaning.

As a social worker I have witnessed what happens when people give up. There are seniors who have tasted much emotional pain and turmoil. Of these, some are unable to accept their lives. Feelings of rejection and loneliness are evident, but no one seems to care. Some feel pressure surrounding them. They feel deprived and that they are without opportunities to improve their lives. Thoughts and fears of dying become prevalent. Some are suicidal. Financial dependency and anxiety over money are distressing realities for many. Their appearance becomes sloppy and personal grooming is neglected. Interest in cooking a meal fades. Gradual deterioration sets in.

Some of the blame lies with society. Dignity, a significant personal value, is often threatened by the economic hardships faced by some seniors and, ultimately, it is up to society, the society which these older citizens supported for so many years, to be helpful by improving their economic well-being. Society must assist them to restore their dignity.

Changes and Their Effects

When some amelioration takes place through an outside source or sources, then values can and often do return to the lives of depressed people. If an older person's health is not too far gone, incentives can be reintroduced. Occasionally, when an older person is depressed, an effort to communicate with a neighbor or friend can be helpful. Visits to a senior center can have beneficial results. Receptionists on duty assist in an initial interview to make a person who is depressed or lonely feel comfortable. Follow-ups automatically ensue. There is a deep consciousness on the part of senior center staff people to lend assistance.

Specific Values Respondents Mentioned

In review, I found variation in how often certain values were referred to. Those most frequently mentioned were:

spirituality	adjustment to change
happiness	knowledge
faith	contentment
perseverance	adherence to ideals and
understanding	principles

Other values that seemed to stand out were:

courage	constitutional determination or fortitude
friendship	
education	self-discovery
love	a sense of humor
hope	unselfishness

Further Ways Values Can Influence Us

Personal experiences guide us. Through them we can improve the choices we make. Due to the complexities of life and the unexpected events that occur daily, we have the opportunity to look into ourselves to understand exactly what is taking place within us. As a result, *new* values can and do spring up.

We cannot simply choose values out of a hat. *They have to be a part of us* before they develop meaning. They must *be developed to be realized.* Many values do not last unless we do something about them. When we are motivated to keep going, there are certain values or ideals which are involved. A sifting of values goes on, more or less, all through our lives.

Personal values can influence us in another way. They contribute to improved physical adjustments. The mind affects the body. When we reflect on society's attitudes toward aging, where seniors often are deposited by the wayside, then personal values frequently can come to the rescue and become a boon, *strengthening our own resolve,* and aiding our ability to cope physically.

Discarding Some Values and Taking On New Ones

Each of us has a hierarchy of values that changes in importance from time to time. Being older need not prevent us from making changes or modifications. Influences causing the changes emanate from society as well as from ourselves.

We usually do not give our values too much conscious thought. They stand like fence posts, guiding us down a particular path. Yet taking the time to think about what we value gives us renewal and a measure of added confidence. Values reflect thoughts and feelings as well as a way of life. They give us power; need we be afraid of this power?

The seniors who hold up best in their later years are those who have values that have been useful and satisfying. Relationships are known to improve by values partners hold.

Avis D. Carlson, in her book, *In the Fullness of Time,* observes this fact:

As I have tried to point out, there are values to be had from old age; real, undeniable pluses. In our society they don't hit us over the head. We have to seek them out, think about them, and put them to the test of practice. But they exist, and they can be sought.

Perspective

Seniors *should* concentrate on what is paramount to them and seek to find fulfillment from the acquisition of the things they value. Such a pursuit can result in great satisfaction.

Every phase of a culture involves values. Values are a key factor in all people's lives. It is therefore fitting that we should become more conscious of the personal and social values that we have chosen to cultivate. A system of values is part of every adult's life, regardless of age. Though we may have limited energy as we grow older, softening our convictions, *values* can still be a source of hope. They can still help us to understand ourselves better and to grow in the process. Understanding breeds acceptance; we can only grow to like ourselves better, which means that ultimately we will grow closer to those around us as well.

Chapter VII
Mental Health

Thought is the seed of action.
—Ralph Waldo Emerson
Society and Solitude

Fortunately analysis is not the only way to resolve inner conflicts. Life itself still remains a very effective therapist.
—Karen Horney
Our Inner Conflicts

How people feel is a critical factor in their ability to be productive. Any effort to promote good health must also include a conscious desire to develop a positive mental outlook. The two go together. Health *attitudes* make us care more about ourselves in general. They improve our expectations. It is the attitude, the frame of mind, that carries us forward.

Attitude is associated with life expectancy. Living conditions, nutrition, and proper medical care are all factors in life expectancy, but attitude controls the will, and the will regulates our ability to do what is good for us. Constructive thinking is vital. If we project apathy and negative thoughts, we shall eventually deteriorate. Research bears this out. Our appearance can affect how we feel, for example. It is known that a well-groomed appearance makes us feel better.

During a group discussion at a senior center, the facilitator set up two headings on a blackboard. There were about a dozen seniors, mostly women of varying ages past sixty-five. They were asked to give their impressions of *Feeling Old* and *Not Feeling Old.* These were the results:

Conditions and Attitudes Associated With

Feeling Old	Not Feeling Old
deterioration	enthusiasm
apathy	positive outlook on life
negativity	agility
unproductiveness	interests
senility	optimism
consciousness of wrinkles	happiness
lack of motivation	loving kindness
	vibrancy

In another senior center, I set up the same two headings on a blackboard with a rap group consisting of about seventeen men. To encourage spontaneity, I limited the time for response to twenty minutes (we ran over about five minutes). Here are the results:

Conditions and Attitudes Associated With

Feeling Old	Not Feeling Old
feelings of inadequacy	enjoyment of retirement
physical deterioration	good health
fears (many kinds)	sexual appetite
loss of self-esteem	physical fitness
feelings of limitation	youthful mental attitude
	adventurousness
	no *feelings* of being old

Not Feeling Old
working
impulse to travel
feelings of freedom
involvement

Interestingly, the men's group dwelled more on the "Not Feeling Old" category, reflecting a preoccupation with the positive aspects of living. A point that was brought up by one of the men was that "society makes seniors feel old by perpetuating false and negative attitudes about age that not only affect how older people are treated, but also how they treat themselves." This group later emphasized that we have to feel good about ourselves, that our self-image is all-important. We should ask ourselves who we are and what image we have of ourselves. Such questioning may enable us to become more the person we would like to be.

Our Mental Attitudes

All people have certain attributes and desirable qualities that should not be wasted. We must learn to bring out the goodness we hold inside by sharing our experiences and trying to understand each other. The ability to communicate in many directions is possible only if we are open with one another. We need not feel limited; the attitude we possess will ultimately determine whether or not we can do something or accomplish our goals.

I initiated another kind of inquiry touching on attitudes during a men's senior citizen rap group. One man stated,

"Time may be running out [the topic]; probably I won't be able to fulfill my ambitions and dreams." The respondents were between sixty-five and eighty-two years of age, but most were in their early seventies.

Of the twenty men present, eight contended that they no longer hoped to accomplish any new goals; several felt that they had lived a full life already and were content to live out whatever time is left to them.

Several men stated that they prefer living in the present and therefore couldn't accurately judge what awaits them down the road (what lies ahead). They believe in the *now,* not in the future, or for that matter, the past.

Most of the group expressed concern over the desire to have continued good health. "Health is a critical factor in being able to fulfill ambitions," said one man who felt, at seventy-three, as if he had accomplished about eighty percent of his life plans. Some of the others desired to continue with volunteer work or other efforts that would enable them to be useful and helpful.

A few members of this group said they have no thought that time is running out on them. Instead, their focus is the satisfaction they're experiencing at present, the joyful memories of the past events, and the overall sense of accomplishment they feel when looking back over the years: communicating well in their marriages, reading and other leisure activities, not having to worry about making a living—these are the things which bring contentment to these men. As one of them pointed out, "Everything is attitude. There are people much younger than anyone here who truly believe that time is running out on them."

Thoughts Shared by My Respondents

"If you don't have the right thoughts, your health can be affected. I think pretty well of myself. I don't disparage myself."

"Your state of mind controls your health."

"I never want anything to conquer me."

"I like my life with happiness and youngness."

Ella, a woman past seventy-eight, said, "A good mental outlook is important—never give up. This consists of having good thoughts and not depreciating oneself, having good food habits, developing positive attitudes, and using one's intelligence." She added that the good habits established in her early life are what keeps her going now.

Gertrude, a former Christian Science nurse in her late sixties, offered some provocative thoughts. She said:

> Age is a crystallization of thoughts. We need to melt, to be forgiving like a child. Never hold resentments. It is our thoughts that put the label on us. We must feel love and give love; see the beauty instead of the ugliness. We should have the beautiful things all of our lives. We should bring heaven to earth. We are never going to take it with us. We all desire greater and bigger things and we have the capacity to obtain them. By our later years we should begin to get a hold of life. Man is here to discover himself (surface—no depth in some people). Awakening is the important thing, not the calendar years.

This last sentence is especially significant for people who feel old.

I have found that achievement makes people happy. If we love ourselves more, we can more readily love others. Can we say that our seniors are in charge of their own attitudes? Or is society in control? Earlier, society may have dictated values to some, but this becomes less and less true in later years. With certain exceptions, older adults tend to take more of a stand in their values and attitudes, becoming more inclined to voice their opinions. These are methods which form positive mental attitudes as one ages. These people are more inclined to be open to expression and "lay it on the line." They show a willingness to seize the initiative and make things happen. These older adults show a vital concern for their own needs.

Here are methods used by some older people to form positive mental attitudes on aging:

"The question of survival keeps me going."

"People are looking ahead to the year 2000. We have to look forward to something—*pleasant, important, significant,* or *worthwhile*" [emphasis mine].

"We tend to put up barriers in communication. The more we know, the more we have obligations to our knowledge."

"Some are blessed with so many things, but they never see them."

"People hold back. You have to give. It's the most wonderful thing to do. We should not copy other people—just be yourself."

"The whole world has got to learn to love. Many times we know what we ought to do, but we don't do it. Some don't have the push."

Blind in one eye, having lost all of her five children, most of them in infancy, Clair, at seventy-nine, said: "I am grateful to hear my thoughts. That's the way we grow from our experiences. You learn that when you're left alone."

My thoughts go to the senior who once told me that people "should grow along with the world." This is an absolute necessity if one wants to maintain a positive mental outlook. Adjustments and readjustments are vital in life, to our environment as well as to changing social and economic patterns. Outwardly, it seems that those who can take more responsibility for themselves can more readily grow along with the world.

Activity Adds to Health

Basic to the subject of mental health is the desire to strive for *continued* good health. Some older adults say that outdoor recreation has contributed to their longer years. Of the factors that contribute to longer life, they give recreation a high priority. Many say the best way to keep well is to keep busy. It is obvious that activity adds to health, physical and mental.

An observation of Simone de Beauvoir, in *The Coming of Age,* is most meaningful:

> The mind and body are very closely linked. For a man to carry out the work of re-adapting a deteriorated organism of the outside world, he must have retained his pleasure in living. And it works in the other direction: good health encourages the survival of emotional and intellectual interests.

Today there is an abundance of medical research to show that the mind can exert a positive impact on the body. Research is also showing that there are new possibilities and potentialities in developing the brain in the older years. Put another way—physical exercise helps the mental development of older people.

In my theme—What keeps you going?—I observed that among those of my respondents whom I came to know quite well, the traits of assertiveness and feelings of self-worth seemed to have a positive influences and, in turn, reflected feelings of well-being. Also, it appears that mental activity keeps the person functioning longer.

Nora, a seventy-six-year-old with a heart condition and poor circulation, illustrates the point that de Beauvoir was making: "I don't feel sorry for myself and lie around and cry. I don't want to deteriorate like my body, with age." Because she likes to be productive, she discovered that she's artistically inclined and now paints landscapes.

Limited in walking, James, at seventy-seven, said: "I think every person can look forward to something good out of life. They should. We don't appreciate life. I don't see anything bad in anybody." He added that he has no enemies. "It's the best feeling on earth."

Jennie, at eighty, belonged to a senior recreation club. She commented, "I am a realist. I take things as they come." Mary, eighty-eight years old, said, "Some people let their minds dwell on themselves too much when they get older. I do not have time to think about myself. Some people have too much self-pity. I am tough or I wouldn't have lived so long."

Another energetic little woman I met as she was just turning ninety-four told me with an air of serendipity, "I don't know how come I am here, but I am still getting around." Kathleen, a spry ninety-eight-year-old Irish lady, gave insight as to why she has been able to carry on so long and still manage by herself in an apartment: "I know how to live or else I wouldn't have lived to this age. I am happy—that is why I have lived so long. I am a happy person."

"I feel that I have a lot of living to do, things that I want to do. I can't give up. I won't give up," stated the active, eighty-year-old Ellen. She is a songwriter and pianist, and volunteers her time in senior centers, convalescent homes, and hospitals. "Laughter is the best medicine in the world for people," Ellen told me. Her philosophy is to "get busy sharing what you have with others. Then you will reap." She added, "Some seniors conduct themselves as though they had a veil over their faces. If they lift the veil, they would see so much more."

I frequently made home visits in my social work. Harriet, ninety-six years old, could still dress herself without assistance. She enjoyed working with flowers. She remarked, "I was well my whole life." Her son verified that his mother is mentally at peace with herself. He said, "A factor contributing to her longevity is that she was deeply concerned with her immediate neighborhood and those around her, and was not much interested in the larger world about her."

Nutrition

Mental attitude is one of the keys to what keeps us going. Mental attitude is often governed by what we eat. A handful of these older adults indicated they keep going because of good nutrition. Nutritional problems are significant in the lives of many older people, presenting obstacles in maintaining a healthy outlook.

Many older people do not place enough emphasis on the importance of eating properly. Yet, giving attention to a healthy diet and foods that have nutritional content is a key to improved healthful living. The standards older people hold are, in part, dependent on economic factors. A lot of older adults feel that, with good nutritional knowledge, they can eat properly on a limited budget. However, a low income often results in poor eating habits. Society plays a part in this problem and should continue to help seek solutions.

A Reader's Digest publication, *Eat Better, Live Better: A Common Sense Guide to Nutrition and Good Health,* states:

> A healthy diet for an older person in good health differs very little from that at any other age. However, moderation in portion sizes may be in order, and particular attention is necessary to make sure that the foods chosen are high in the protective nutrients—protein, vitamins, and minerals—since many older people are less active than they were in earlier life. To cope with reduced appetite, the older person might have nutritious snacks in addition to three smaller meals daily. . .

I highly recommend this guide. Its contents touch on the "ABC's of nutrition," being quite informative. For example, it indicates that studies have shown that overweight is more often caused by a lack of exercise than by overeating.

Frequently we older persons give the excuse that we are too old for exercise. This brings to my mind the January 7, 1992 *Los Angeles Times* article, "Keeping Fit," wherein an eighty-one-year-old man, Bill Selvin, was featured. Selvin is the founder and executive director of Growing Old Gracefully, Inc., based in Irvine, Orange County, California.

The article states, "He is dedicated to exercise programs for senior citizens and is trying to enlist an army of assistants to help spread the word." Selvin has already received some funding. The article mentions that he "doesn't pull any punches," and quotes Selvin as saying:

> I tell people the less activity you have and the less you move your body, the sooner you're going to your grave. If you want to die in a hurry, it's easy. Just do nothing. Sit in a chair, watch TV, and go to the refrigerator during every commercial. (Copyright, 1992, Los Angeles Times. Reprinted by permission.)

Another excuse many use is, "I'm too tired to exercise," as though exercise will exhaust them. The Reader's Digest guide states, "On the contrary, exercise relieves fatigue, stress, and tensions."

Often publications advise people that, when getting up in years, their exercise must not be excessive. It is advisable before starting an exercise program to obtain a doctor's approval, especially if one has not been physically active for years.

The combination of good nutrition and exercise go together for well-being and health. Our mental attitude is also interlaced with these factors. For instance, I found it interesting that those of my respondents who referred to *having good nutrition seemed more likely to have social contacts than those who didn't.* A few were married. Those not living with a spouse frequently did not eat alone; they reached out to others. This illustrates a point noted in the Reader's Digest guide:

> Nothing stimulates care in preparation of food, not to mention actual appetite, like the prospect of company. Many nutritional ailments are symptomatic not just of poor diet but of poor social contact . . . [A]n elderly nutritionist advises attending to loneliness first, then the diet. *Those who believe they have a future, and a stake in present health, will make a greater effort to participate in life by caring for themselves through diet* [emphasis mine].

Further Use of Capabilities

"One needs challenges and the stimulus of ambition all through life," commented Lillian, a well-read woman of seventy-nine. This certainly is a way to keep going. We must accept challenges. To face new challenges, one might fight fear. It's well worth the effort. When we do away with fears, our general health improves and we can face challenges more easily.

Many older adults speak of having their ups and downs, testifying that life is not always at an even keel.

In a workshop for seniors entitled, "Emotional Ups and Downs," someone pointed out that people have nothing to gain from feeling down; if we try to learn from every situation we are in, then there is no way to stay down. When we're down, we have a different perspective; we wish to find an "out," a means of turning the tables. We try to bring about ways to accomplish this change. As a panelist said, "We have a lot of living to do." Life always poses a challenge.

A woman in the group, now age sixty-eight, said that she has at least twenty more "long years" left, and that many diverse interests will fill up her time. A woman in her fifties added, "Reasoning that I have the power to make things happen has contributed to obtaining nice things, paving the way for them to happen."

Another senior group discussed the topic of living in the present. Some of the comments were:

"Looking forward instead of backward keeps me going."

"I am not necessarily giving too much thought to what will happen, but *living with hope each day*" [emphasis mine].

Norman Cousins, in his *Anatomy of an Illness,* notes:

> . . . long before my own serious illness, I became convinced that creativity, the will to live, hope, faith, and love have biochemical significance and contribute strongly to healing, to well-being. The positive emotions are life-giving experiences.

A force within must emerge to bring to surface the emotions and feelings of which Cousins speaks. It takes a considerable amount of intense effort and concentration to reach such a point.

Some years ago, in my fifties, I suffered a bronchial condition with a wracking cough. I felt that I was a "goner." After more than a week, some improvement took place. Unexpectedly, I became conscious of the trees I could see from the windows of my home. The deep green of nature made a profound impression on me. I was alive to enjoy this scene—I was most grateful. Filled with the very feelings Cousins speaks of, I had survived. When life is threatened, it's easier to see the healing potential of all things around us.

Having a Purpose

To keep going, take a stand. Find a pursuit that is satisfying. We need goals to attain our objectives. *Purposes can be of many kinds, and they should give some drive and ambition to the person.* Any purpose in life may change to some extent as the person grows older. My respondents have shown many kinds of purposes. Their minds and sensitivities are opened by the impact of their purposes.

A Mental Attitude: Believing in Ourselves

It is important to plant the thought that we, as older people, are useful, that *we are valuable in our own right.* This is not an exaggerated perception. Such thoughts can genuinely motivate us to keep going. We cannot think of ourselves as small and limited human beings. Nothing external can dictate what sort of people we should be. We can blossom at our own pace, and as we see fit to do so. When we retire, our feelings about ourselves should not diminish. In fact, the extra time at our fingertips can call us to improve our stature. In retirement, we have the opportunity to become more useful to ourselves and to those around us.

Occasionally, we are able to say, *"I am stronger than I thought I was."* We shouldn't sell ourselves short. I had the pleasure of visiting a lively lady named Ida, age eighty-six, residing in a retirement home. Along with two other senior guests, she entertained us with a rendition of "Dark Eyes" on her cello. I was impressed with the spirited musician's coordination and movement. Our cellist friend said that she likes to keep busy and to feel she's accomplishing something. She had mentioned having the desire to perform once again with other musicians in an orchestra. Being able to turn people on at an older age by showing some kind of artistic ability can be magnetic. Additionally, the appreciation shown by those present had left a happy imprint on the performer.

I learned that Ida had raised two children and had been a secretary for many years in civil service. She had always been outgoing with a sense of humor and was always the life of the party. In her sixties, Ida joined a symphony orchestra, playing the cello, which she continued for many years. Ida was active till the very end, recently passing away at age ninety-two.

Here is an interesting passage from the book, *It Takes a Long Time to Become Young,* by the playwright Garson Kanin:

In her seventies, Marlene Dietrich continued to draw sold-out houses everywhere in the world. She said: "They don't come to see me just because I take the trouble to look as good as I can. They come because I represent something—courage, stamina, faith, motherhood, who knows? Sometimes they just sit there in stunned silence, amazed that I'm still alive and moving."

Perhaps some of what Marlene Dietrich represents to her audiences can be incorporated into all of our lives in varying degrees.

How We Can Have More Control of Our Lives

The desire to better understand ourselves and take action can have rewards. We may develop more control over our lives. Yet, there are no prescribed methods for the way different adjustments are made.

If we encounter resistance from various sources while trying to lead a better life, we can try to be more assertive. We must act with *boldness* and *courage.* Trying to understand what we feel can help. Adversity, sorrow, and grief can lend additional inner strength to help us achieve a more satisfying life.

In counseling sessions that I have attended, the advice has been consistent: *"Don't deny your feelings."* This is a good plan to live by. Allowing feelings to come out in the open aids in developing more peace of mind and more serenity from within, but like everything worthwhile, it takes effort.

I met Laura in a senior camp setting where there were many kinds of social activities being offered. At sixty-five, she shows continued growth. As she made these statements her eyes lit up, mirroring her deep convictions:

> You have to use your mind, to move, to live, to laugh, or to die on the vine of life. I will think as long as I can think. I will move as long as I can move. I will thank God that I am able to use myself as long as I can. I live by a day to day philosophy. Now that I am retired, for the first time in my life, I have time for me. Freedom is the most exciting thing to have in every sense of the word, to come and go, to do as I choose, to be able to say: "I choose to do!"

Donald, an eighty-four-year-old, offered some good advice: "Live an honest life. Look at the bright side. Push your trouble back behind you. Worrying just upsets your whole system and it'll make you sick."

We all experience our advanced years differently, depending on such factors as environment, emotional growth, income, education, and the religious beliefs we have had. We seek avenues to circumvent the noticeable slowing, to prevent emotional turmoil, and lessen physical deterioration. Any effort to find ways which will help stave off these problems will be well worthwhile. We all have many unexplored thoughts and feelings that need to be sifted out and decided upon.

Pausing Briefly to Reflect

I wish to convey to my readers some good techniques on relaxation. When we are tense, we miss what is going on about us. The soul needs to *quiet down* to enable us to enjoy and observe what life can hold. *A quiet state of mind* is desirable in order to fully benefit from the beauty that surrounds us. We have to take time to relax, to pause a while, and we need to be in pleasant surroundings whenever possible. A smile, a touch, a caress, a kind word, a compliment—all add to relaxation. We must take time regularly for these; we must make time for the beauty that is all around us.

Lucky is the senior who can wonder about things like a child. The more we gear ourselves to wonder, the more we shall be able to explore. There is a child living in every one of us, and it needs recognition. Children frequently can let go of their feelings without effort. In our older years, many of us can benefit by these positive influences. Just watch the spontaneity of a child when giggling or laughing! This turns us on, and we cannot help but also smile.

Contact with children in our older years can add a stimulus to our lives. We can gain much by identifying with children's natural curiosity. This is a tremendous trait they have. How to explain the questions they ask! What inquisitiveness! Being receptive to their inquiries lends much to grandparent and child relationships. I consider myself fortunate in that I have three grandchildren, the oldest being five and a half. My grandchildren's overt responses are so natural and warm, framing an added dimension to my life. We should never give up this childlike curiosity in our older years.

An expert on an educational TV program relating to "kids" stated, "They understand better when they are doing something." I like this point and feel it is appropriate to people of any age. I become impressed when I turn to Helen Keller's remark about never losing her "childhood sense of wonderment." In the *Speaker's Treasury of Anecdotes About the Famous,* James C. Hume cites a meaningful passage:

> On her eightieth birthday, Helen Keller was asked, "How do you hope to approach 'old age'?" Characteristically, she gave the classic reply: "One should never count the years—one should instead count his interests. I have kept young trying never to lose my childhood sense of wonderment. I am glad I still have a vivid curiosity about the world I live in. And so, I think I'm still as young as my interests." . . .

In the pursuit of new interests and growth, it is surprising how many directions we can take. Our choices are practically unlimited. They exist in such diverse areas as social interactions—including relationships with the opposite sex—work objectives, taking further educational courses, or developing a greater interest in books, theater, or music. The idea is to promote what talents we have and to also explore new areas. It simply takes a measure of decisiveness and strength of purpose to get started. Most of us sell ourselves short.

We should regularly visualize the things we wish to have in our lives. Then we must act on these dreams, turning them into goals. Dwelling on our limitations is not the answer. If we desire something special, we must set our minds on it. Knowing what will keep us going evolves from knowing what we want. Then we must make a sort of contract with ourselves.

Being a happy and successful senior stems from having

a positive outlook, but cultivating such an approach to life takes time and effort. A positive attitude results from a gradual and steady way of thinking for those who are willing to make the commitment. Each day can be a new beginning, and tomorrow can be a promise of hope.

More on Attitudes

Katherine, an energetic person, one month shy of ninety, said, "I never thought of age." She explained that she was a "doer" and found it hard to be on the other side of the fence at her age. She mentioned having been interviewed by a local newspaper three years earlier, expressing herself well with a delightful sense of humor. The subject of a burial plot came up in another instance. "Death is about the last thing I think of. I have the energy and get-up for the whole family," exclaimed one eighty-eight-year-old woman.

I spent the better part of an hour with ninety-eight-year-old Henry, and his nephew, in Henry's home. The nephew said, "My uncle has a strong constitutional determination." This conveys that Henry has strong physical and mental attributes, and is not easily sidetracked. He has a resoluteness and persists against discouragement.

Three Final Comments on Well-Being

"I am thankful for the gift of life."

"If you can give to someone else, you have an eye on life."

"I try to keep myself healthy, to keep going."

Chapter VIII
Seeking Gains in Ourselves

A man is not old as long as he is seeking something.
—Jean Rostand

When we do the best we can, we never know what miracle is wrought in our life, or in the life of another.
—Helen Keller
Out of the Darkness

What are possible ways to bring about gains in ourselves? At times it is not easy for the older person to search his or her soul to find ways to deal with deep feelings. But this effort is often greatly rewarding. Those who volunteered to express their feelings on this book's theme seem to have the following qualities:

A point of view
A sense of direction
An identity
Hope

Many seniors have these traits. Those who don't can attain them. It simply takes work. Limited contentment, lack of fulfillment, or feelings of restlessness can drive us on to new accomplishments. At age ninety, the famous pianist Artur Rubenstein declared, "I will never give in."

Some abilities increase with age. For example, the aptitude for statesmanship, medical research, literature, invention, exploration, conservation, and astrophysics, to name a few.

Seeds of Maturity

Joe Denhart recently addressed the subjects of maturity (and immaturity) in his class "Aspects of Living," for older adults. Denhart teaches this class as part of Glendale Community College in Montrose, California.

He attributed maturity to people who:

learn from their mistakes
have suffered
are not perfect
are getting "seasoned"
have characteristics of love, joy, responsibility, and
   integrity.

Maturity points to mental competence and is an ongoing process. It doesn't mean perfection.

Along with the above traits are:

patience
an even temper
acceptance
ability to deal with reality

    ability to exercise good judgment
    self-control
    compassion
    common sense
    flexibility
    ability to learn from experiences
    ability to be nonjudgmental
    ability to solve a problem as it occurs

Do these traits strike a chord in you? You might possibly have many of these. Each of us would prefer to have a mature outlook. My respondents, regardless of age, showed varying levels of maturity.

As Denhart stated, mature persons have the qualities of love, joy, and integrity. These traits were evident among a number of my respondents. Many displayed other traits on the above lists such as dealing with reality, having compassion, being sincere, and learning from their experiences.

Keeping mindful of the above traits, we can think more about the word "maturity." Every day is a new beginning when our minds focus in this way. It is a way of getting our emotional needs met. These needs can be contentment, gratitude, and ability to give to others, for example. Also, *we need one another.* We can be self-sufficient, but should not take it to an extreme.

Even if the word "maturity" is not in our minds, we older adults are ever mindful of the concept. For instance: Who hasn't learned something from their mistakes, or hasn't suffered in some manner, or has not shown some kind of love, joy, or responsibility? In daily routine living, our good traits often go unnoticed, but we should allow them to see daylight. In Denhart's class, some of these were brought to focus. It is stimulating to review what may be distinctly inside of us and what we may take for granted.

Learning to feel good about ourselves and accepting ourselves should be our highest goals. More awareness and intensity of living can help us reach these goals. All through life, we try to seek further gains with ourselves. In whatever manner, something drives us toward further improvement and understanding.

Some Ways to Carry On

It is therapeutic to discuss why we continue with our lives. We review our past and, by using what we've learned from our experiences, we can improve our attitudes and values. We tend to search and find the best within ourselves. The project is endless. We can literally continue each new week with new thoughts.

Occasionally, when seniors are asked how they are *coming along,* they will tersely reply, "I am surviving." The answer is vague, as though they were not clear as to which direction they were heading. Asking what keeps them going, however, usually brings forth responses which reflect more foundation, more thoughtfulness.

Here are some brief answers from a senior group when asked, "What keeps you going?"

"A thread of hope."
"A miracle of some sort."
"Love (all kinds)."
"To get new ideas from other people."

"Curiosity."
"I have much to do."
"I am motivated."
"To have an interest in life."
"I want to discover my pluses."

I was affected by a news article I read where an older couple was planning a vacation, and the wife remarked that they may be taking a trip for the *last time.* Her feelings made me pause and reflect.

The possibility that we may be seeing or doing something for the *last time* should make us appreciate fully what we are now experiencing. Drive, curiosity, and an urge to give more to life are often results of pausing to look at our existence and of wondering *how much longer* we have on earth. As for myself, feeling that life is short, I take more time now to remind myself what friendships mean to me, what the walks I take through old trails, forests, and the countryside are worth, and how much I value my visits with my two sons, who live in another state.

At times it takes a strong jolt, such as the sudden loss of a friend or significant remark, to bring about a change in our outlook. Adversity, as discussed in a previous chapter, can be a steppingstone to change. Growth comes from suffering.

The Importance of Remaining Open

Richard Kalish, in a book he co-authored with Lillian Dangott, *A Time to Enjoy: The Pleasures of Aging,* illustrated the idea of remaining open. He discussed the effect a woman in her mid-seventies had on him. He met her in the Sierra Mountains at an elevation of about 10,000 feet.

> She walked slowly, using a cane but, walking with her, I found myself thoroughly enjoying her special enthusiasm and curiosity. This woman, in her extraordinary openness to new experiences, changed my whole perspective on life and aging. That people can continue to grow now seems obvious to me. They can continue to live excitingly, to develop potential *at any age* [his emphasis]. Until I met this woman, I assumed that old age was all grief and no joy—and I dreaded it.

This writer's reaction demonstrates how easily our attitudes can change if we merely keep ourselves open.

Seniors often express a need for stimulation and incentive. Many older people are eager for change. They are open to new experiences. A man in his seventies said, "Life is beckoning me onward." In a news interview, eighty-year-old Abner Kreisberg, a dean of American numismatics (the study of coin collecting), pointed out, "The main thing to do is keep your mind active. Otherwise you disintegrate." When we examine our feelings, we are less likely to remain complacent.

Conversation often places a person in the limelight—an appealing position for the person getting on in years. We hold more tenaciously onto life when we share it with others. Talking brings out mutually beneficial anecdotes and past events.

In a rerun of an interview on KCET, Corporation for Public Broadcasting, the late Norman Cousins said, "The important thing is what we do while we're alive. The great tragedy of life is not death, but what dies inside of us while we live." He further stated, "Precious life is being wasted.... New thinking and new hopes are being born.... We should give a pretty good account of ourselves while we are here."

In a retirement newsletter I receive I found these words: "Don't worry about failure. Worry about the chances you miss when you don't even try." Norman Vincent Peale stated, "Several studies have found that people with a positive sense of themselves will work harder and longer, and that, in turn, their perseverance allows them to do better.... And if the mind thinks with a believing attitude, we can do amazing things."

I raise these questions: What can we do to improve our functioning? Do we try to be in touch with ourselves? Where should most of our energies go? What more can we do to learn from our setbacks, our adversity, our pain?

I have come away feeling that a positive thought or idea, whatever it may be, can suddenly take effect on someone who has previously been filled with negativity, and can strongly influence that person to take positive steps toward personal improvement. To continue developing incentives in the older years; to feel that life continuously has meaning; to always radiate confidence; to endeavor to function reasonably well physically; to have interests that remain with us; to feel that we are loved, that people care about us—not to feel alone, and to never have thoughts of giving up—all these can make our lives buoyant and livable.

Adversity contains the seeds of opportunity. Frequently, the limitations in our midst goad us to improve what we potentially have—to learn more, to strive more, to face problems with more resolve. Just one or two successes can pave the way for more. We can improve our inner qualities. For example, our potential can be expressed in writing. Possibly, we have accumulated ideas that could be set down for others to see and appreciate. The idea is to find what we continue to like to do, *and do it!* We need to develop feelings of contentment, *feelings of well being, as we expel our superficial self-image.*

Adjustments made after retirement are most rewarding. They take intense effort; *they take action.* Attitude makes the difference. For some, changes in this area will be necessary, but changing our consciousness can begin by a simple change in our routines. Writing down our goals and other positive statements will help.

Taking stock of our assets makes us aware of available resources. Can we give ourselves encouragement? Do we take the initiative? Can we motivate ourselves into action? If we are resourceful, we shall be able to deal effectively with difficulties. At intervals problems will arise, but we must simply confront these difficulties in order to overcome them. Too frequently we limit ourselves. Our eyes are closed to opportunities.

If we examine our environment more closely, we will find "extras," enabling us to develop more hope and confidence and, at the same time, higher expectations. It is a matter of adding interesting things to our lives. If we don't succeed in a certain endeavor, then we can try alternatives. We can ask ourselves, What next? The sum of our experiences can lend direction and guidance. Spiritual insight can also be a key.

We should put enthusiasm into whatever we do. A

nonagenarian put it this way, "If you look forward to what you are doing, enthusiasm will keep you going." It is *having something to do,* keeping occupied, that counts. Enjoyment of life takes root when we push ourselves into action. Involvement is the answer. We should try to be in control of our lives as long as possible. There is no age limit on what people can do with their minds. *Make more of what is left of life.* As one senior has said: "Aging is the refusal to shift your life into neutral."

Priorities are a way to go. Priorities lend a spark to our lives no matter how old we are. They stimulate us to keep moving, lending more meaning to our existence. We should ask ourselves now and then, What are our priorities? What concerns us now most? What do we wish to get into? What might be a second prospect? And so on down the line. In short, we should ask ourselves where we shall turn our energies. We need to set priorities.

Adding to people's lives reflects one of my priorities. This priority resulted in this book. The more security I could feel within myself, the more I could reach out and contribute to others.

By our efforts to communicate, we are not permitting isolation to set in. It's the contacts made with others that lend perspective to who we really are. In a lifetime, the interaction with others also aids in our keep-going journey.

In seeking gains, do we give reasonable time and thought to our families, giving them a feeling we care? Do we try to stay in touch with world events and developments? Are we able to incorporate values that relate to friendship, compassion, humility, and other worthy values?

Eda Le Shan in her book, *Oh! To Be 50 Again* observes: "When we accept the changes we see in ourselves we can begin to make vital and exciting choices for ourselves." Acceptance of self, coupled with action, makes us able to continue facing life. It takes strength to offer what we know. We have more attributes than we are willing to believe. Each person has something substantial *to tell,* or *to do.* There are many stories never told, feelings never expressed, and abilities never shown—literally a tragic waste. It's a never-ending process to know who we are.

Chapter IX
In Summary

I would like to express several deep motivating factors which compelled me to write this book. I enjoy warm contacts with people. This is a special kind of fulfillment for me. Certain human contacts and settings were prominent in my life.

Two teachers in particular stirred me into a pattern of research. Forty years ago, I had taken several sociology courses with Dr. Harold T. Diehl, a professor with whom I had much rapport. While standing outside the classroom during a "break," we touched on my career plans. I told him that I was interested in the field of social work. Looking at me squarely, he replied in a strong, measured voice, "You're a researcher!" His exclamation made a significant impression upon me. He said research in sociology was a way to go. Dr. Diehl's response carried over all through the years, always remaining with me. I learned never to underestimate this quality he felt I had.

Another teacher who influenced me was Dr. Ann Morgan Barron, whom I met about thirty years ago. She was a speech teacher and therapist who also dealt with problems relating to geriatrics. She was already up in years herself. I not only learned speech methods in her class, but I also developed much in common with her dealing with seniors.

In those early years of delving into senior concerns, Dr. Barron was very instrumental in organizing a group called Gerontological Leaders, Inc., of California. In this organization, for the time it functioned, I learned more about the general needs of our older population and what we considered were legislative priorities. There was also the pleasure of meeting and collaborating with a number of dedicated people in the field of aging.

Dr. Barron liked my concerns with older generational needs. At that time, she suggested I apply for community adult-education teaching. Not having sufficient hearing to qualify, I was turned down. Wearing hearing aids was not recognized at that time. The end results, of course, disappointed me. This teacher's passing not too long after left a void within me. She left a legacy that imbued me with a desire to take up the needs and aspirations of our senior adults. Dr. Ann Barron was a pioneer in the field of aging. This fact, coupled with her distinguished qualities, left deep impressions on those who had come to know her.

Both these teachers were important people in my life. I became more dedicated by knowing them. They helped ingrain in me a spirit to strive and contribute, in the remaining years left to me, to the older population.

The last motivating factor I'd like to mention is my employment (not long after Dr. Barron's passing) as a research coordinator (later termed "research consultant") with the Los Angeles County Department of Senior Citizens' Affairs. I assisted in initiating, at one point, a questionnaire given to all Los Angeles' incorporated cities. The questionnaire was part of "Services to Seniors," as the Department was in the process of further developing plans for the retirement years of all L.A. County's older population.

"The focus on helping the older person stay involved in the total life of the community" was the intent of the Board of Supervisors by way of our Department of Senior Citizens Affairs. Assisting in coordinating the results of this survey made a decided impact upon me. The survey was influential in my becoming more involved with older people and their varied problems, strivings and aspirations.

After my work retirement, I became preoccupied with the theme of "Keeping Going." It is my hope that I have increased practical knowledge relating to gaining more control over our lives. I also hope I have stimulated a desire for thinking and activity along these pathways. Promoting more understanding in what older adults feel, and their concerns, are of primary importance in the field of aging and the greater society.

I have pointed out that there is insufficient recognition given to the fact older persons are capable of making meaningful adjustments after retirement. This book speaks to older adults with no specific support system to lend opportunities for growth. With my respondents' presentations and other information in this book, I have tried to show it is possible to create a more positive aging in our society.

Possibly some of the insights here could result in some kind of policy on a national scale. We could gather a much larger number of respondents' views on what keeps them going and publicize the results nationwide. Conceivably, our seniors could develop an expanded vitality. The overall gains may not be immediately evident. Aging represents challenges. We need to search for practical knowledge which may benefit our older citizens.

The world-at-large must be more informed.

I have given many suggestions and encouragement to older adults in the Activities and Personal Interests chapters in ways to be mentally as well as physically active. Increased leisure time demands adjustments.

An inner faith voiced by respondents contributes to their mental attitudes, as reflected in the Mental Health chapter. In view that a system of values is part of every adult's life, regardless of age, the Personal Values chapter reflects the benefits gained from various kinds of values held.

When entering into the chapter of Family, Friends, and Lovers, we turn to discussions in promoting relationships, expressing feelings, living purposefully, and, in general, making adjustments.

In this book, I've attempted to discover more about the never-ending process of who we, as older adults, are. Many older adults develop certain realistic outlooks as to where they stand, and it shows. The goodness of their thoughts and beliefs show. "What keeps you going?" is a fundamental question that can be addressed to anyone, and generally brings interesting replies.

I have attempted to shed more light on the things which motivate us in our older years. Developing positive attitudes is important. In each chapter, I've stressed the need for positive attitudes. Inner faith is necessary to move toward these attitudes. Respondents have given their own conceptions of what they want for themselves. By absorbing what these people are seeking for the remainder of their lives, we may learn valuable lessons of our own. These adults touch on many facets of living, and they produce many answers.

In the main, previous generations of older adults did not discuss their innermost feelings. More older adults are voicing their personal needs and opinions with less restraint, when given the opportunity. With proper encouragement, more of their feelings will surface. This will be relevant in shaping their future as well as that of the greater society. People from other countries of the world could also benefit from these developments. With the trend toward a longer life span, more people can aim for further usefulness and achievement.

Efforts to improve health and to pursue activities such as hobbies, volunteerism, adult educational programs, and good relations with family and friends will result in greater feelings of well-being. If you permit yourself, you can directly benefit.

By reflecting on what has been pictured in my book, can it be said that a person might have better control over his or her life? My answer is "Yes!" As we have seen, there are multiple ways for seniors to remain motivated. Recognizing that we have distinct feelings and hold valuable and unique answers should brighten each of our lives. We need only to get in touch with ourselves, and then share our discoveries with others.

We can imagine life as a journey; we are forever moving, and it behooves us to put some spark into the process. Along the way, we should bite into life, keep our curiosity, and never allow ourselves to stagnate. We must put something into the "kitty" of life to make any future gains. I am not speaking of the far-distant future. These respondents' various insights reflect an ability to tap into a foreseeable future. They have developed certain guidelines that lend a solid base. This is not a panacea, something unreachable. We should believe in something, have a course to follow. The future does not have to be remote.

Let us all move on to further experiences and *maximize* our older years—make every day count. Why not concentrate on the person you are right now and make new beginnings? Life is precious, and we owe it to ourselves to make the best of it. Let's do it. We pave the way for the future to come to life—our own future!

Bibliography

Andrus, Ethel Percy. *Power of Years.* Long Beach, California: NRTA and AARP, 1968.

Bengston, Vern L. "Research Perspectives on Intergenerational Interaction." In P. Ragan, ed., *Aging Parents.* Los Angeles, California: University of Southern California Press, 1979.

Beauvoir, Simone de. *The Coming of Age.* New York: Warner Books, 1973.

Blanton, Smiley, M.D. *Love or Perish.* New York: Simon & Schuster, 1956.

Butler, Robert N., M.D. *Why Survive?* New York: Harper & Row, 1975.

Caprio, Dr. Frank S. *Add Life to Your Years.* Secaucus, New Jersey: The Citadel Press, 1975.

Carlson, Avis D. *In the Fullness of Time.* Chicago: Henry Regney, 1977.

Case, Clarence Marsh. *Essays on Social Values.* Los Angeles: The University of Southern California Press, 1944.

Cebotarev, Dimitri. Director, Soviet Union's Institute of Gerontology. "The Right to Old Age." United Nations Headquarters: New York, 1971.

Colton, Helen. *The Gift of Touch: How Physical Contact Improves Communication, Pleasure and Health.* New York: Putnam, 1983.

Corly, Nan, and Judy Maes Zarit. "The Unmarried Later Life." *Sexuality in the Later Years.* Ed. Ruth B. Weg. Academic Press: San Diego, 1983.

Cousins, Norman. *Anatomy of an Illness.* New York: W.W. Norton, 1979.

Croft, Roy. "Love." In *The Best Loved Poems of the American People.* Ed. Hazel Felleman. Garden City, New York: Garden City Publishing Co., 1936.

Dangott, Lillian R. and Richard A. Kalish. *A Time to Enjoy the Pleasures of Aging.* Englewood Cliffs, New Jersey: Prentice-Hall, 1979.

Denis, Ruth St. Qtd. in Howard Whitman. *A Brighter Later Life.* Englewood Cliffs, New Jersey: Prentice-Hall, 1961.

Douglas, Dr. Richard. University of Michigan Institute of Gerontology. Qtd. in Carol Stocker and Martin F. Kohn, "Some People So Good at Being Old." *Star-News.* Pasadena, California, Jan 1979. Reprinted by permission of Richard Douglas.

Downs, Hugh. *Thirty Dirty Lies About Old.* Niles, Illinois: Argus Communications, 1979.

Dubos, Rene. Qtd. in Morton Puner. *Getting the Most out of Your Fifties.* New York: Crown, 1977.

Feingold, S. Norman. *The Futurist.* World Future Society, Bethesda, Maryland, July/August 1991. Reproduced with permission from *The Futurist,* published by the World Future Society, 7910 Woodmont Avenue, Suite 450, Bethesda, Maryland 20814, (301) 656-8274.

Gardner, Joseph L. *Eat Better, Live Better: A Commonsense Guide to Nutrition and Good Health.* Ed. Joseph L. Gardner. Contributing Writers, Robert Bahr, et al. Pleasantville, New York: Reader's Digest Association, 1982.

Greeley, Andrew M. *Faithful Attraction: Discovering Intimacy, Love, and Fidelity in American Marriage.* Tom Doherty Associates, New York, 1991.

Harris, Louis. "Who the Senior Citizens Really Are." Address at the Annual Meeting of Council on the Aging. Sheraton-Cadillac Hotel, Detroit, Michigan. October 2, 1974. Photocopy: 3.

Hepner, Harry W. *Retirement—A Time to Live Anew.* New York: McGraw Hill, 1969.

Hirsch, K., & Linn, M.W. (1977), "How Being Helpful Helps the Elderly." *The Gerontologist,* 17(5) Part II, 75, October 1977 (Abstract).

Hume, James C. *Speaker's Treasury of Anecdotes About the Famous.* New York: Harper & Row, 1978.

Kessler, Julia Braun. *Getting Even with Getting Old.* Chicago, Illinois: Nelson-Hall, 1980.

Kuhn, Maggie. Qtd. in "Twelve Perspectives in Living" in E. Jane Oyer & Herbert J. Oyer, eds. *What Really Matters.* Brattleboro, Vermont: The Stephen Greene Press, 1981.

Marriot Corporation International Headquarters. "The Marriot Seniors Volunteer Study." Commissioned by Marriot Senior Living Services and United States Administration on Aging. Marriot Senior Living Services, Washington, D.C. April 1991.

Marsh, DeLoss L. *Retirement Careers: Combining the Best of Work & Leisure.* Charlotte, Vermont: Williamson Publishing, 1991.

Maslow, Abraham H. *The Farther Reaches of Human Nature.* New York: The Viking Press, 1971.

Maslow, Abraham H. "New Knowledge in Human Values." In Titus. *Living Issues in Philosophy,* New York: American Book Co., 1964.

May, Siegmund H. *The Crowning Years.* New York: J.B. Lippincott Co., 1968.

Mechanic D. "Social Factors Affecting the Mental Health of the Elderly." *Mental Health of the Elderly.* Eds. H. Hafner, G. Moscnel, N. Sartorius. New York: Springer-Verlag, 1986.

Mulac, Margaret. *Leisure Time for Living—and Retirement.* New York: Harper & Brothers, 1961.

Raths, Louis E., Merrill Harmin and Sidney Simon. *Values and Teaching: Working with Values in the Classroom.* Columbus, Ohio: Charles E. Merrill Publishing Co., 1966.

Reedy, Margaret Neiswender. "What Happens to Love? Love, Sexuality, and Aging." *Sexuality and Aging.* Ed. Robert L. Soinick. Ethel Percy Andrus Gerontology Center, USC, 1978.

Roosevelt, Eleanor. *You Learn by Living.* New York: Harper & Brothers, 1960.

Rubin, Theodore Isaac. *Real Love, What It is and How to Find It.* New York: Continuum, 1990.

Sanderson, Jim. "Affection—Especially at Age 75." *Liberated Male.* Column in *Los Angeles Times.* Part V, Sunday, August 3, 1980.

Schaie, K. Warner, and Geiwitz, James. *Adult Development and Aging.* Boston: Little, Brown, 1982.

Sidransky, Ruth. *In Silence: Growing Up Hearing in a Deaf World.* New York: St. Martin's Press, 1990.

Simon, Sidney B., Leland W. Howe, and Howard Kirshenbaum. *Values Clarification.* New York: Hart, 1972.
Titus, Harold H. *Living Issues in Philosophy.* New York: American Book Co., 1964.
Trueblood, Elton D. "The Blessings of Maturity." *The Courage to Grow Old.* Ed. Phillip L. Berman. New York: Ballantine Books, 1989.
Vischer, A.L. *On Growing Old.* Boston: Houghton Mifflin, 1967.
Walbroehl, Gordon S., M.D. "Educating Elderly Patients About Sex." *Geriatric Consultant.* Ed. John Lavin. Medical Publishing Enterprises, Fairlawn, N.J. May/June 1990.
Weg, Ruth B. "The Physiology of Sexuality in Aging." *Sexuality and Aging.* Ed. Robert L. Solnick. Ethel Percy Andrus Gerontology Center, USC, 1978.
White, Dr. Paul Dudley. Qtd. in Morton Puner. *Getting the Most Out of Your Fifties.* New York: Crown, 1977.